SAVING SIGHT

SAVING SIGHT

An eye surgeon's look
at life behind the mask and
the heroes who changed
the way we see

ANDREW LAM, M.D.

IRIE
BOOKS

Irie Books
12699 Cristi Way
Bokeelia, Florida 33922
sales@AndrewLamMD.com

Author's Note
The names of patients and healthcare providers, and some aspects of the cases described in this book, have been changed to protect privacy. Some passages in this book are dramatized accounts of true events.

Cover and author photos by Baystate Health
Cover and interior design by Mariah Fox, ital art

ISBN 10: 1-61720-379-3
ISBN 13: 978-1-61720-379-4

First Edition
10 9 8 7 6 5 4 3 2 1

To Alex, Audrey, Sophia, and Daniel

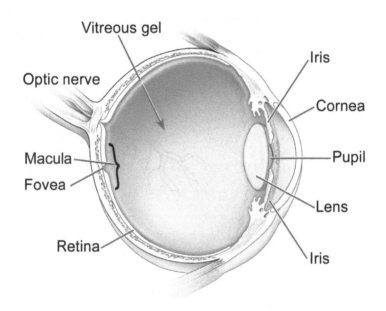

A cross-section of the eye
viewed from above.

*Courtesy of the National Eye Institute,
National Institutes of Health.*

CONTENTS

Chapter One | **LUCKY**

I was still outside, but I could hear her yelling.

"I knew something like this would happen! Why'd you tell him to go work at that place? Why?"

They were an African American couple, huddled close at the center of the deserted hospital lobby.

Glass doors slid apart and I walked in from a cold, dark December night in Philadelphia.

"Do you realize he's gonna be BLIND?" the woman shouted.

I couldn't keep myself from looking. She was petite. Little clumps of unmelted snow lined the furrows between her tightly braided cornrows. Her harsh stare bore into the chastened man, and now, up close, I could see the tears running down her cheeks.

"Why'd they let him use that machine? Didn't he wear safety

glasses? Oh my God! My son's gonna be *blind!*"

Even at a distance, her diatribe made the few people in the Emergency Room's waiting area cringe. I cringed too, because now I knew this woman's son was the one I had been called in to see.

I entered the treatment area and steeled myself.

Our hospital was an *eye* hospital, and our Emergency Room was one of the few in the country solely dedicated to eye care. Normally, the scene inside was hectic, with nurses trotting back and forth and residents rushing between rooms or to the phone to accept referrals from outside hospitals. And even when it wasn't crowded with patients, there was always an energetic vibe about the place, buoyed by the upbeat nurses and a close camaraderie among residents who labored through the intense training program together.

This time, however, everything was different.

The space was deathly still and silent, except for the isolated shouts of the mother in the lobby. The door to exam room two was shut. Madeline, a wise-cracking nurse in her sixties who'd worked here for years and seen all manner of horrific eye injuries, now looked serious and sullen. She glanced at me sympathetically as she walked by.

"Hi Andrew, thanks for coming," said Theresa, the first year ophthalmology resident. Her hair was disheveled. I could tell she was tired from being on duty for over twelve hours already.

"What's going on?"

"It looks really bad…" She pointed to the closed door. "Auto mechanic. Definitely ruptured."

I sighed. It was late on a Saturday night. I was not going to get much sleep.

"How?"

"He was grinding metal. No safety glasses."

I nodded. Behind me I heard Madeline call the patient's parents in from the lobby. She took them into room two and closed the door, which did little to mute the sound of the mother's exclamations. She was really upset. I was about to enter a lion's den.

I knocked, opened the door. Jacob was a stocky twenty-four year old. His name was stitched onto an oval patch affixed to the chest of his gray, grease-stained overalls. I couldn't see his face at first because he was bent forward in the exam chair, moaning quietly. I came closer. Rivulets of blood and tears ran down his cheek from under the plastic shield that had been taped over his right eye.

"Hello everyone. I'm Doctor Lam, the retina fellow." I'd already completed my ophthalmology residency but was in the middle of specialty training for retinal surgery.

The woman grasped my outstretched hand. *"Please,* save my son's eye," she pleaded. Even though there was an extra chair, the father stood in one corner with his arms tightly crossed and his shoulders drawn in as if bracing himself for a grenade blast.

"I'm very sorry we're having to meet like this," I said, turning to Jacob. "I understand you were hit in the eye with a piece of metal this afternoon. Let me take a look and see what's going on."

I gently removed the shield and immediately saw that the right eye was ruptured. It looked like a squashed grape.

"Jacob, I'm going to check your vision now."

He struggled to open his eyelids a little. "It's really dark, Doc."

"Let's just see what it is." I covered his good eye and held two fingers in front of his face. "Can you see how many fingers I'm holding up?"

Jacob shook his head.

I waved my hand in front of him.

"Can you see my hand moving?"

He squinted, then nodded. "I can see a shadow moving."

I sat down facing him and carefully positioned his head into the frame of a table-mounted microscope called a slit lamp. I gently opened his lids and looked through the scope.

Oh no.

At first I thought the cornea was missing. All I saw was a black blob mixed with some dark brown iris tissue. Had the contents of the eye been expulsed? I'd never seen that before, but I knew it could happen if the patient coughed violently or vomited while his eye was ruptured like this.

I drew a deep breath and looked closer. *Wait.* Now I could make out the torn edges of a huge laceration, starting in the center of the cornea and extending laterally, beyond the edge of the cornea and into the sclera. How far back did it go? I couldn't tell; it was a bloody mess. The normally white sclera and conjunctiva of the eye were torn, swollen, and beefy red. I realized the dark blob in the center was mostly clotted blood. It was impossible to see the lens or anything else in the back of the eye.

Can this eye be saved?

I wasn't optimistic.

"Did you happen to find the piece of metal that hit you?" I asked. "I mean, was it a big piece that might have bounced off, or a tiny piece that could have gone into the eye?"

There was an uncomfortable moment of silence.

"Well, what was it?" the mother abruptly lashed out. Her husband winced. He was shorter than his son, with "Elvis" sideburns and a receding hairline. Staring at the floor, he muttered, "I don't know. I didn't see it. I didn't look."

The mother threw up her hands and groaned.

The father looked at me with quiet, desperate eyes. "Do you need me to go back and try to find it?"

"Don't worry about it. We'll get a CT scan to see if there's anything in the eye now."

I answered some of their questions and went back out to make sure Theresa had started antibiotics and anti-nausea medications.

Forty-five minutes later, we slapped the CT films up on the light box. In the middle of the eye cavity, on practically every cut of the scan, there was a large reflective object, shining bright like an exploding supernova. A child could have diagnosed it. The metal was still in the eye. I didn't see a posterior exit wound, damage to the optic nerve, or any brain injury.

Can this eye be saved? I asked myself again. Nine out of ten ophthalmologists would have probably said, *No, don't even bother trying to put it back together. Just go straight to enucleation.* Removing the eye entirely would eliminate the risk of *sympathetic ophthalmia,* a rare inflammatory condition in which severe trauma to one eye induces the body's immune system to attack the fellow eye. *Plus, artificial eyes look so good these days,* many might say. It's true that a prosthetic eye would probably look far better than whatever I might be able to do with Jacob's shredded eye. No one would fault me for telling the resident to call in the oculoplastic surgeon to remove the eye. Enucleation was almost inevitable in cases like this. I could be home and back in bed in less than an hour.

Except that we were at the famous *Wills Eye Hospital.* The nation's first eye hospital and the institution of last resort for countless patients. The culture of the place was to *always* try to save the eye. If nothing else, this would give Jacob some time to psychologically prepare for the loss of his eye.

Except that this was probably the worst rupture I'd ever seen.

I went back in to talk to the family.

"Jacob has a ruptured eyeball," I told them. "The metal is still in there. I've got to be honest, I'm not sure we can save this eye – " The mother gasped. I slid closer to her and put my hand on her shoulder. "But we're willing to try. We can do a surgery tonight to try to remove the metal and sew up the wound. I promise we'll do everything we can."

The mother cried softly as I patted her shoulder, thinking it odd to be comforting her while her injured son sat in stoic silence. Then I thought about how I would feel if my son was about to go into surgery, against long odds, and we sat there, all of us, in silence for a while.

Before I left Jacob said only one other thing. "I trust you, Doc.

Thanks for helping me."

An hour later, I stood over him as the anesthesiologist inserted a tube down his throat for general anesthesia. I started having doubts. *There's no way I can salvage this eye. It's like a bullet hit it dead on. The iris, lens, retina – it's all going to be torn up inside.* I began to think of all the ways Jacob's life would be altered after losing one of his eyes. He'd be tentative about playing sports for fear that his good eye might get injured. He'd always have trouble with depth perception. He wouldn't be qualified to drive a truck or a school bus. Was he married? I didn't know. For some reason I wondered if his scarred, sightless eye would reduce his confidence with women.

He was ready. The ruptured eye was exposed – a bundle of scrambled tissue and blood – the rest of the field covered by a blue drape. I blinked hard. Time to go to work.

To determine the full extent of the laceration, I dissected the conjunctiva to expose the scleral part of the wound. I breathed a sigh of relief when I saw that it stopped about three millimeters beyond the edge of the cornea and had not affected the insertion of the lateral eye muscle, which was still attached.

My first goal was to get the metal out. To do it, I'd have to be able to see through the pupil into the back of the eye, so I squirted a steady stream of saline though the corneal laceration to wash out the dark, clotted blood. I began to see the iris. It was torn in one area, but most of the pupil still looked round and intact. The lens wasn't so lucky, I could see it now. Instead of being clear, it was cloudy, almost opaque, with fluffs of lens material emanating from a gouge in the center of the lens capsule.

Traumatic cataract.

I wondered how an episode of *CSI* might illustrate the moment of impact: a jagged metal piece flying toward the eye in slow motion, bursting through the cornea, knifing through the lens, and ricocheting toward the retina in the back of the eye. Then they might show a retinal detachment or an avulsed optic nerve or half a dozen other blinding injuries that, if they were real, would make this surgery a long, futile exercise. *CSI* would make it interesting and cool. But this was *real*. This was Jacob. A nice, hard-working guy whose parents loved him and who had a long life ahead. I inserted the instrument ports that would allow me to access the inside of the eye and wondered what I was going to find.

Though it pained me to do it, since Jacob was so young, I knew his damaged lens – his *cataract* – would have to come out to enable me to see into the back of the eye. Everyone gets cataracts if they live long enough. When this clouding of the lens begins to interfere with vision the cataract can be surgically removed and replaced with an artificial lens. This usually happens to people when they reach their seventies or eighties. I was going to have to take out Jacob's lens at twenty-four.

I inserted an ultrasonic probe into the eye. Controlling it with a foot pedal, I emulsified the lens and sucked it out. A young person's lens is soft and this cataract came out easily in a few minutes.

Now I could see that the middle of the eye was full of blood, which was mixed with the sticky vitreous gel – the clear substance that normally fills the eye. I let out a sigh and realized how tensely I had been flexing the muscles in my neck. I tried to relax.

Slowly, carefully, I began to remove the blood using a *vitrector* – a thin probe with an opening at the tip and a blade inside to cut up and suck out the blood and vitreous. The view was murky. I prayed that I wasn't inadvertently chewing up a detached retina. And, I didn't know when or where I'd come face to face with the piece of metal.

Finally, I got a glimpse of the retina, specifically the macula, which is the most important part of the retina and subserves central vision. *It probably hit here,* I thought, because the macula lines the rearmost part of the eye.

To my surprise, the macula looked okay. The optic nerve, too.

There was no sign of the metal fragment.

As I cleared more blood, I began to see ugly, jagged, criss-crossing white scars beneath the retina. These were areas where the concussive impact of the projectile had ruptured the choroid, the layer beneath the retina. *Wait.* One of these scars wasn't just a scar. It was a huge retinal tear. *Uh-oh.*

But where's the metal?

I could almost see the whole retina now. The tear worried me, but I had to stay focused on finding the foreign body. After slicing through the lens, the fragment must have deflected downward and crashed into the retina. As I pictured this, the beam of my light probe glinted off something shiny.

The metal.

It looked huge in my view through the operating microscope. Jagged, at least five millimeters across. It was lying on a bed of bruised retina, looking like a meteor that had just cratered the moon.

How the hell am I going to get this out?

It was too big for forceps. No intraocular forceps would have jaws that opened wide enough. There was a special basket-like instrument for scooping BBs out of the eye, but this shard was too oddly shaped to use that. And what if I *could* grab it? Normally, we'd remove foreign bodies through one of the nice, neat scleral incisions I'd already made to insert my instruments into the eye. Sometimes we'd have to extend the incision a little bit to accommodate a bigger foreign body, but this? This was too big. I'd have to slice open an entire quadrant of the eye to get this out.

There was only one way: to take it out the way it had gone in, through the gaping wound in the front of the eye.

"Get the magnet," I told my assistant.

The magnet was a long, thin metal probe, which I carefully inserted into the eye. Trouble was, this magnet was designed to extract much smaller and lighter pieces of metal, nothing like this monstrosity. Would it be strong enough to pull out this piece?

I advanced slowly, closer and closer to the metal.

Nothing was happening.

Was it broken? How long had it been since someone had used this?

Years?

I was almost touching the fragment when I saw it tremble, then shift, and then stick to the tip of the magnet.

Whew.

I lifted it gingerly; it was a tenuous hold. I tried to push the metal up through the pupil and into the front of the eye. It wobbled, I froze. I tried again, but it got snagged on the iris. I advanced and snagged, advanced and almost lost the hold, advanced and then finally got it past the iris, only to bump into the edges of the corneal laceration. With my other hand, I passed forceps through the wound to grasp an edge of the piece, but I couldn't get a grip. Then, suddenly – I gasped – the metal came off the tip and fell back into the eye.

No!

Had it just landed on the retina and caused more damage? Another crater?

I quickly found it again inside the eye. Fortunately, the macula still looked okay. I thanked God that I'd put in perfluoron®, a heavy viscous liquid, to cover the macula and cushion the impact of any falling fragments.

But now what?

I went over my options. I could try again, but the same thing might happen and I couldn't be sure the perfluoron would save me again. I could get a stronger magnet. This one would be a lot bigger, the size of a toothpaste tube, with a pointy tip that I could put at the entry wound; but, I wouldn't be able to insert it *into* the eye, and it was so strong that the metal would fly rapidly at it with great force. I'd have no way to control the fragment, which would probably damage the iris on its way to the magnet. A final option was to cut open a big swath of the sclera and take it out that way.

By now the top of my mask was damp with sweat. The surgery was taking a long time, and the OR was strangely silent. Everyone knew that all the work I had done before had been for this moment. The surgical assistant, circulating nurse, and anesthesiologist were all watching closely. Like me, they desperately wanted Jacob's eye to be saved.

I decided to try again with the probe magnet.

This time I asked my assistant to help me spread the wound open a little wider by lifting up one edge of the cornea with forceps. I went in with the magnet and slowly drew up the metal. I got it past the iris again and into the anterior chamber of the eye. The magnet was barely holding on. *Don't drop it, don't drop it,* I prayed. In my other hand, I had a light probe inserted into the eye. Now, in one make-it-or-break-it move, I pushed the piece up and out with both the magnet and light probe, trying to shove the metal through the wound.

The fragment disappeared.

"What just happened?" I said aloud.

I stared at the magnet in my hand. It was now protruding out the front of the eye. There was nothing on it.

Dropped again?

I quickly looked back inside the eye.

No metal.

Where is it?

"Wait!" my assistant shouted. She pointed into the pool of blood-tinged saline that had collected in the drape pocket next to the eye. I shined my light probe. There was something shiny.

And there it was. We scooped it out. Now, with the naked eye, it looked pathetically small. I didn't care. I breathed a sigh of relief. *We got it.*

There was still a lot to do, but nothing as nerve-racking as what I'd already done. I used a laser probe to encircle the big retinal tear with laser burns that would help prevent the retina from detaching. I carefully sewed the two edges of cornea and sclera back together. It took a while, and in the end the repair looked like a long seam of baseball stitches, but it was sealed and water-tight.

When I'd finally finished, I tried to stand up and almost fell over because my legs were numb from being in the same position for so long. I stumbled off to the side, letting the nurses and anesthesia team recover the patient. I ripped off my mask and took a deep breath. I'd done everything I could. I hoped it was enough.

—

The eye freaks a lot of people out. Come at the eye with something as simple as an eye dropper and some patients lurch back, or worse, faint. Medical students are often no better. Most of my classmates wouldn't have dreamed of going into ophthalmology. As a whole, they might be as likely as my twin seven-year-old girls to think that working on the eyeball is just plain gross. Furthermore, most medical students get the idea that being a doctor requires having a stethoscope draped around your neck, a tool you'd be hard-pressed to find in an eye surgeon's office.

So it's no surprise that a lot of doctors consider ophthalmology a fringe specialty. An orphan. These days, many medical schools don't require students to have *any* clinical training in ophthalmology. With everything else in medicine growing more complicated, with so much else to learn, there seems to be no time for it. And yet, the complexity of eye diseases and ocular surgery demands at least four years of post-medical school training to master. And when any of us develops a sight-threatening eye problem, the first thing we do is search out the best-trained eye doctor around.

I may be in the minority, but I've always thought the eye is cool. To me, it's the most amazing organ of the body – a perfectly designed device whose delicate parts act in concert to help us perceive and make sense of our world, do our work, appreciate beauty. I chose to be an ophthalmologist. After four years of medical school, I did a one-year internship, a three-year residency, and a two-year fellowship to sub-specialize in retinal surgery. That's a lot of years, but it didn't feel like a burden. Along the way I kept learning more and more about the eye, and the more I learned, the more fascinated I became. It wasn't hard to convince myself that going into ophthalmology was one of the best decisions I'd ever made. So many of the treatments were quick, effective, and often delivered dramatic results. We could take out a cataract and replace it with an artificial lens in under fifteen minutes. We could repair the retina, the delicate, gossamer neural tissue that lines the inside of the eye, and bring back the sight of patients who'd just gone legally blind from a retinal detachment. Today, ophthalmologists use lasers to correct refractive errors (a.k.a. LASIK), transplant corneas, and implant retinal chips to enable blind people to read letters and navigate a room. It's always difficult to speak objectively about the present, but I'm confident future physicians will look back and say that I am practicing during a golden age of ophthalmology.

The better I got at diagnosing and treating diseases, and the more adept I became at operating, the more curious I grew about how our current techniques had developed. Who had come up with this machine that sucks the cataract out of the eye with such ease? Who had dreamed that we could put an artificial lens in the eye? Come to think of it, who had figured out *how* to look at the inside of the eye in the first place?

As I learned more about the history of our field, I was continuously struck by two marvelous facts. First, only a mere thirty or forty years ago, well within our lifetimes, hardly any of the treatments I regularly perform today had been discovered. Ophthalmology, like many specialties, lay fallow in a kind of dark ages. But as medical knowledge and technical innovation increased, the development of new treatments exploded. This type of growth happened in other fields, too, but the revolution in ophthalmology was truly remarkable.

The second thing that amazed me was that most of these advances were made by a few individuals. Just regular eye docs. They weren't the big-shot, big-name giants of the field. In fact, those academic, establishment types were more often guilty of hindering the young innovators who were challenging the status quo with their new ideas. No, the doctors whose inventions have benefited millions of people weren't famous, and they weren't even geniuses. They didn't have parents who'd given them a leg up in the field. They were people whose dedication, persistence, ingenuity, and luck, brought them success. The stories I was unearthing were incredible; the trials these innovators endured sometimes bordered on the unbelievable. That we would arrive where we are today was never a certainty. It wasn't inevitable.

Even though the advances I'm talking about are less than three decades old, and in some cases occurred while I was training in the 2000's, I soon realized that I was learning about history, without thinking about it as historical. Like a lot of Americans, I love history. I've observed that we are exceptionally proud of our own history. We treasure and preserve places as obscure as the tiny Philadelphia townhouse where Thaddeus Kosciuszko lived for a few months after the Revolutionary War (it's the smallest unit of the National Park Service). We hallow isolated plots of land like Monocacy, Maryland, where a little-known battle was fought during the Civil War. I've seen the battlements of Normandy, the ruins of Pompeii, and the terra cotta warriors of Xian, and I never failed to wonder how much better we might protect these treasures if they resided in America.

But then I've also thought, if Americans love history, why do we know so little about the heroes I was reading about, people whose work has saved the sight of millions around the world? Their biographies could be made into blockbuster Hollywood movies. Most of us have heard of a few medical icons – like Pasteur, Jenner, or Salk – but compared to the detailed attention we pay to professional athletes and movie stars, we know very little. And the real-life heroes of the eye are nearly forgotten – by all but a few curious ophthalmologists who chat about them over dinner at their annual meetings.

I began to feel almost honor-bound to share their stories, if only so that young people might learn what "ordinary" people can achieve. I wanted everyone to know about these medical heroes who didn't make it onto the cover of any magazines and whose neighbors probably never knew they were living next to someone "important."

The pages of this book will transport you into the past and share the journeys taken by the heroes of ophthalmology. Along the way I'll also share what it's like to progress from naïve medical student to skilled retina surgeon. I'll explain why practicing medicine today isn't exactly how I'd pictured it would be, because our decisions are too often defensive rather than curative, driven by fear of litigation and sometimes financial gain, or, worst of all, indifference because of vast amounts of paperwork and hassle. And yet, there is always the fundamental fulfillment that comes from saving and improving vision. I am often amazed by my patients, who will do anything to save their sight – whether it's to undergo surgery, have needles repeatedly stuck into their eyes, or take half a dozen eye drops every day for the rest of their lives if we tell them to. I've hugged men who wept out of gratitude for regained sight and embraced others whose descent into blindness made them suicidal.

Always, every single day, I appreciate what those who came before me dreamed, discovered, and suffered to enable me, and doctors like me, to save sight today.

—

Jacob's eye healed relatively well after his surgery. Despite the odds, he got to keep his eye, with vision good enough to count fingers at one foot.

No one would claim that this level of vision was very good. If I was making this story up, I might say that he had a miraculous recovery: 20/20 vision, after a corneal transplant and an artificial lens. But this is real life, and real life – so far – doesn't work that way.

But then again, sometimes real life can inspire in ways that fiction never would. Like the way Jacob thanked me in the early days right after his surgery, and the gratitude he felt for the chance to keep his eye. He didn't wallow in self-pity for the vision he'd lost.

He felt lucky.

Chapter Two | *"This operation should never be done."*

HAROLD RIDLEY AND THE INTRAOCULAR LENS

I scanned the chart quickly on my way to the exam room.

Ms. Rodriguez. Fifty-nine years old. From Puerto Rico, Spanish-speaking only.

Ms. Rodriguez was heavy, with a neck that seemed to be a continuation of her chin and a few folds of belly that peeked out from under her shirt. When I entered the room, she was staring blankly at the floor.

I know just enough Spanish to be enthusiastic.

"Hola, me llamo Dr. Lam! Como esta?" I spouted, wearing a big smile.

But Ms. Rodriguez's expression didn't change. The heavy lids of her downcast eyes didn't move. Was she sleeping? I thought she might be. But then her shoulders rose and fell as she heaved a slow breath, and I looked closer. She was awake, but she looked despondent, like her dog had just died.

"Hello, Doctor," came a young woman's voice from the corner of the room. I turned and blinked. Her daughter was stunningly beautiful – like Jennifer Lopez, right here in the room with me. But she wasn't happy, either. There was no spark in her eyes, just – exhaustion?

A young man, the patient's son, was seated near the sink. He sat quietly, expressionless, giving off a vague negative aura, as if this was the last place he wanted to be. He flinched away from the water as I washed my hands even though no drops came anywhere near him.

I exchanged a few pleasantries with the daughter, who spoke English. Then I looked closer at the chart. The technician's note said Ms. Rodriguez's vision was limited to "counting fingers" in both eyes, which meant she could see one or two fingers if you held them a few inches from her face. She wasn't able to read the big "E" on the eye chart. Under *Previous Eye History* was noted a "lazy" left eye from childhood, a term some patients use to describe *amblyopia* – the vision in that eye had never developed. Under the box headed *Last Eye Exam* was written, "Never?"

I asked the daughter a few questions. Her mother had been a seamstress all her life, but she'd been unable to work for at least three years. Her vision was so bad that she could no longer read or even see images on the television. For three years, she'd spent her days in bed or on the couch doing nothing, depressed and possibly suicidal, to the point that her children took turns staying with her overnight, each taking a week at a time, while they held down their own jobs – she at a nail salon, he as a security guard.

All of this information came from the daughter, who seemed worn out but also hopeful. The son remained silent and grim. Perhaps he was against seeing doctors, and maybe that's why his mom had never seen an eye doctor? Or maybe he thought I was too young to be a surgeon? Maybe he was just bored.

I examined Ms. Rodriguez. Both eyes had very dense cataracts. A cataract forms when the lens, which focuses the light rays entering the eye to a point on the retina, becomes cloudy and opaque. Think of the eye as a camera. The glass at the front of a camera is akin to the eye's dome-shaped cornea. The human lens is similar to the camera lens, and the retina is like the film in the camera. Ms. Rodriguez's cataracts were mostly of the *posterior subcapsular* variety, which means there was a dense frosting on the back surface of her lenses. These are the most visually-debilitating kind of cataracts, and now I understood why she could only see counting fingers.

The cataracts also clouded my view inside her eyes. Although I could tell the retinas were flat and not detached, it was too hazy to gauge the health of the optic nerves, which connect the eye to the brain, or the maculas, the most important part of each retina because they subserve central vision.

I informed the family that she was a candidate for cataract surgery in the right eye. It wouldn't be appropriate to operate on the amblyopic, "lazy" left eye, because even with the cataract removed, we couldn't expect it to see well since it had never developed normal vision. I was a resident – still in training – so there would be an "attending" surgeon supervising me.

They agreed to the surgery.

When you're a resident in a surgical field, you're a lot like an indentured servant. A good resident will work hard to show how earnest he or she is, be quick to help the attending physicians (the bosses) with the smallest tasks, and *always* display fascination at what is being taught or shown. The worst thing a resident can do is have a bad attitude. The second worst thing is to be lazy.

I used to have a fairly cynical view of this system of teaching, particularly in medical school, when I was paying $40,000 a year for the privilege of being someone else's underling. But when I finally got to the point where the attendings were teaching *me* how to operate, my cynicism vanished. You see, from the attending's perspective, teaching a young, inexperienced resident how to perform surgery can be one of the most stressful experiences imaginable. Residents are more likely to cause complications, and attendings assume the ultimate responsibility for each patient's outcome. So it's actually small recompense to play a subservient role out of respect for their willingness to train us.

A week later, I operated on Ms. Rodriguez. Because we knew her other, amblyopic eye had no potential for improved vision, the stakes were high; this would be her only chance to see.

When nothing goes wrong, modern cataract surgery is the most elegant surgery ever devised. It takes ten to fifteen minutes. A diamond blade is used to make a tiny, 2.75 mm wide incision in the peripheral cornea. A small needle with a bent tip is utilized to make a circular hole in the front surface of the lens capsule. An ultrasonic probe is inserted through the tiny incision, through the hole in the lens capsule, and is then activated to break up and suck out the nucleus and cortex of the cataract. Finally, a folded artificial lens is injected into the eye. As it goes in, it unfolds and is positioned in the lens capsule, which was left behind to hold the artificial lens. The surgery is done. The incisions are so small that no sutures are needed.

Thankfully, Ms. Rodriguez's surgery went just like this. Perfectly.

The next day, I walked into the room where Ms. Rodriguez was waiting. Before I could say a word, she leapt out of her chair and cried, "Dios Mio! Gracias!" She hugged me. She kissed my hand. She was crying.

I was stunned. I couldn't believe she could move that fast. I stood there for a moment as she squeezed me tightly, and then I glanced at her chart. Her vision was 20/30, which meant that she could see at twenty feet what a normal person could see at thirty feet. Her son and daughter were beaming. The Jennifer Lopez look-a-like was tearing up and her brother was smiling so hard, I didn't recognize him.

I thanked them and took a look at her eye. The lens was in good position. I expected her vision to improve further once the usual post-operative inflammation subsided, and after new glasses were issued a few weeks later. Her macula and optic nerve looked normal for her age.

In future visits, Ms. Rodriguez remained energetic and happy. She began to read again. She could enjoy TV and go on walks. The exercise helped her to lose fifteen pounds in a few months. Her children no longer had to stay with her, and had no fear she might kill herself. By regaining her sight, she had regained her life.

If you ask any ophthalmologist, he or she will probably be able to tell you a story, or several, of a patient they have helped in almost this exact same way. Cataracts are the leading cause of blindness worldwide, and cataract extraction is the most commonly performed operation in the world. Each year, 1.6 million cataract surgeries are done in the United States, and millions more occur abroad. Rarely has a medical treatment ever been so effective, with such rapid improvement, and at such little risk and cost. Our techniques are so refined that patient expectations are now very high. My own grandfather enjoyed 20/20 vision in his right eye after his first cataract was removed. When the vision in his left eye improved to "only" 20/30 after his second surgery, he was peeved. He asked his doctor what had gone wrong and how he'd "messed it up."

The clear, post-surgery vision that my grandfather and other patients now take for granted was made possible by the invention of one man, Harold Ridley. This quiet, unassuming Londoner invented the artificial intraocular lens. His discovery is legend among ophthalmologists because the inspiration for it originated from a serendipitous encounter between Ridley and a Royal Air Force pilot named Gordon "Mouse" Cleaver during the Battle of Britain. Flight Lieutenant Cleaver earned a place in history by serving his country in war, but because of what Ridley went on to do, his life would take on far greater significance. And now these two men's stories will forever be entwined.

The dramatic narrative that follows is based on fact, but since some details of Cleaver's air battle are lost, and he never published a firsthand account, part of this re-telling is thereby fiction – yet it is fiction that holds to much of what we know is true.

———

RAF Airbase at Tangmere
AUGUST 15, 1940

"Hey Mouse! Bag any?"

Danny, the crewman, slid back the plexiglass canopy of Flight Lieutenant Gordon "Mouse" Cleaver's Hurricane. Danny's straw-colored hair blew in the wind. He was a skinny seventeen-year-old from Manchester.

Mouse cut the engine and slumped back in his seat, beads of sweat pooling at the bottoms of his goggles, which were half-steamed up. He ripped them off and drew a deep breath of fresh air.

He shook his head. "Not this time, old chap. Don't think so, anyway. Perhaps I frightened a few away, at best."

Unlike some pilots, Mouse didn't need to feign bravado. He was already an ace, with seven Germans shot down and two probables. He didn't need to prove himself to anybody.

Mouse staggered out of the cockpit, stretching his sore joints. Warm air blew over his face, and he savored it. Already the cool sweat that had collected in the small of his back was growing hot and sticky here on the ground, so he wrenched off his flight jacket. His goggles were still in his hand. *Damn things.* They always blurred up his vision. He tossed them angrily back into the cockpit. *Up there, seeing the other guy first is more important than anything else…*

"Go get some food while you can," Danny said. "I'll get her

refueled."

Mouse looked at Danny's bright face and nodded. He always looked at Mouse with those admiring eyes. Mouse knew he would give anything to be accepted to flight school. He'd taken the boy up once, in one of the trainers, and even let him have a hand at the controls. Danny was euphoric, the kid looked like he'd just lost his virginity. He had the bug all right, but at the same time Mouse hoped Danny would never learn to fly. Too many old friends gone already.

He started for the large green tent, where ham sandwiches and tea would be waiting. His walk was slow at first, sounding out his legs, cramped after their cockpit confinement. But his stomach growled and he stepped up the pace. To the right, two more Hurricanes cut their engines, one with a badly shot up rudder, but the pilot seemed alright.

Mouse ducked into the tent where he saw Max Aitken, the squadron leader, looking somber seated in a corner, nursing a cup of tea. Mouse walked over to him. Wind-burn and sun on Aitken's normally pale skin around his goggles had produced a funny-looking raccoon-eye tan. A cigarette dangled from his lips.

"How many?" Mouse asked.

Aitken looked up and took a pack of Rothman's out of his top shirt pocket. He tapped out a cigarette for Mouse.

"A few mates still out yet, but so far we've lost five of the twenty."

"Too many. And kills?"

Aitken brightened slightly. "At least seven definites, all Heinkels, and five probables."

"Well, that's something."

Aitken lit Mouse's cigarette for him, then Mouse slumped into a wooden folding chair next to a table with day-old sandwiches on a tin platter. He took a deep drag, then reached out and stuffed half of one into his mouth. The bread was stale, the ham tough. He washed it down with a glass of water an orderly had brought him.

"I can't see how they can keep this up for much longer," Mouse said between bites.

Aitken nodded. The man was never one to sow false optimism. The Luftwaffe had sent hundreds of planes across the Channel for the last two days, many more than usual. The pilots had heard rumors of decrypts that revealed Goering was calling for an all-out attack, code-named *Operation Eagle,* to break the RAF once and for all. Mouse had sortied six times in forty-eight hours.

The two men sat together, chewing sandwiches. A few other pilots did the same, all wearing the same drained expression. Just outside the tent a group of soldiers wearing clean uniforms kept their distance. *Visitors,* Mouse thought morosely. *Here to see what it's all about.*

Suddenly, a shrill whine broke the silence.

The soldiers outside the tent jumped back. Mouse hung his head. The alarm crescendoed. Aitken stood up, and Mouse wearily did the same. He tried to clear his mind, willing the old adrenaline to return.

"Tally ho," Aitken mumbled sarcastically as he broke into a trot toward his plane. Mouse followed.

His Hurricane was exactly where he'd left it.

"Danny! Let's go!"

Danny looked at him, wide-eyed. "Sorry, Sir. Haven't had time to fuel-up."

Hurricanes were already taxiing, taking off. Mouse scanned the field, saw the two new planes, delivered the day before, parked under a camouflage canopy beside a copse of trees.

"Those ready?" he shouted over the roar of engines.

Danny shrugged.

Mouse ran for it. A crewman saw him coming, anticipated what needed to be done and started pulling away the wheel chocks.

"She ready to go?"

"Aye, Sir." This crewman, a short, stocky fellow with a Welsh accent, saluted. "Good hunting, Sir."

Mouse climbed up into the cockpit, noting the shiny new fuselage, the pristine plexiglass canopy. He settled into the seat and realized – *Blast! No goggles.* He'd left them in the other plane. He snapped the canopy shut. *Who cares? I'll see that much clearer in a fight.*

He took the Hurricane out over the grassy field, rumbling, speeding to catch up with the others. He began to feel the familiar excitement build, overcoming his exhaustion.

Time for duty, and to down some Jerries.

Now aloft, the squadron turned toward Dover, twelve Hurricanes, the most they could muster with short turn-around time. Clear of others, Mouse set the button on his control stick to "fire" and tested his guns. The trigger was sensitive – he liked it – and the guns made his stick rattle in an oddly reassuring way. He liked the feel of this new plane, it handled well.

Out ahead of him, he could make out the white cliffs against the grey Channel. Small dots sliding across the sky. Flickers of light in the distance.

Mouse began to climb so he'd come in out of the sun, which still hung a few hours above the western horizon. They were closing now. He could see them, twenty lumbering Heinkel bombers in formation. Me109 fighters flying a few thousand feet above them, yellow-nosed, seeming to hover, waiting to counter-pounce on the attacking Hurricanes.

For a moment, Mouse thought maybe he should continue to climb, take the 109s head on. His eyes flicked from the Heinkel squadron below to the 109s higher up. *When we dive those fighters are sure to bounce us, and take a few of us down.*

But his mates were already screaming toward the bombers. *Well, that's how they trained us.*

He switched on his reflector sight, gritted his teeth, and dove.

The last German bomber was his, its dorsal and waist guns already blazing away. He closed fast. Tracer bullets whizzed past, criss-crossing his field of vision which was now centered on the fuselage of his target. The radio chatter barely touched his concentration.

The bomber's black painted cross grew larger and larger. Mouse tilted forward, fighting the G's, keeping the nose down. He started to angle ahead, estimating where the target would be in ten seconds, seven seconds, five...

Suddenly, his brain registered Aitken's voice, shouting, garbled, over the radio.

"Mouse! Mouse! Jerry's on you! Mouse!"

Small bangs rocked the side of his plane. Mouse felt himself veer off line. He looked right, an Me109 closing fast, now zooming right over him, banking away.

Mouse looked forward again, the bomber was gone, it had passed below him. He'd missed his chance.

He checked the skies. To his left, he recognized William Cresskill's plane, it had a yellow stripe on the tail and ten iron crosses painted on the side. He was the most successful pilot in the squadron. William gave him a small nod. *All business, that chap.*

Suddenly, Cresskill's right wing exploded.

An Me109 screamed past, guns still blazing.

Mouse watched, horrified, as Cresskill's Hurricane broke apart, the tail floating down, the cockpit plummeting and on fire.

Mouse searched the sky for a parachute. *God help him.*

Chatter on his right wing. *Someone's on me!* Mouse jammed hard right; the plane turned and dove. His right aileron was sluggish, but he didn't look at it, didn't look back, already knowing the Messerschmitt was on his six.

Tracers whizzed past. There were impacts behind him, seeming to walk their way forward. His chest tightened, expecting to be shot in the back any second.

The altimeter was spinning, down, down. The ground was close, the trees loomed larger. Mouse didn't dare look back, for fear of hitting the ground. Seconds from crashing, he flattened out and braced himself.

He was most vulnerable now, with the German above and behind, so the hits didn't surprise him – but the shattering canopy did.

In an instant, his eyes were on fire, his vision black. The wind hit his face like he'd run into a wall.

Mouse put the nose up...*climb, climb.*

With his left hand, he fumbled to feel his face.

He realized he was going to die.

The surprise of this occupied his mind for a few seconds. Then his eyes were on fire again, searing, unimaginable pain. It almost made him *want* to die, anything to stop the pain. He prayed the end would be fast, that it wouldn't hurt any more.

He flew like that, climbing blind, for...three seconds? Thirty seconds? He wondered if he'd blacked out.

There's no up or down anymore.

No sense of direction.

Where's the Jerry?

Mouse lifted his arm, feeling for the canopy. It wasn't there. He gripped the stick and put the plane into a roll. Praying he had plenty of altitude, he unbuckled his straps as he turned upside down, and dropped out.

His body was buffeted by a vortex of wind. He spun, head over heels, legs twisting, arms dangling. The sound of the engine was gone, now only wind.

He pulled the cord and felt the sudden gallows jerk. He was flying up, and he imagined himself under water coming up for air.

The ascent stopped; he began to float.

He kept his eyes clamped shut, and tried to remember the landscape.

Farms? Yes, and rolling hills.

Lakes? Ponds?

He didn't remember. A Hurricane flew over three hundred miles per hour, 440 feet per second – it did no good to guess what awaited him, except that it distracted him from his burning eyes.

He hit the ground hard, made worse because he hadn't braced for it. The blow knocked the wind out of him, and everything went black.

Flight Lieutenant Gordon "Mouse" Cleaver was shot down near Winchester, England that day, August 15, the climactic day of the Luftwaffe's *Alderangriff* ("Eagle Attack"), a massive aerial assault intended to cripple Britain's Fighter Command. It was the largest air battle in history to that date, involving over a thousand warplanes.

Mouse had been blinded in both eyes by dozens of plexiglass shards from his shattered canopy, which were now embedded in his eyes. His face was disfigured. He would later undergo eighteen surgeries of the eyes and head.

He was already a hero, one of the very few who saved England from Hitler's invasion in the summer of 1940, but though no one knew it at the time, his greatest contribution to his countrymen, and to humanity, was yet to come. The person who turned Mouse's misfortune into humanity's gain was a soft spoken, unassuming young ophthalmologist named Harold Ridley. He was a relatively short man, five feet, four inches. With his round wire glasses, he had the look of a librarian, or perhaps a zoologist. The thing you notice about older photos of Ridley is that he's not smiling. In fact, he looks downright sad, even depressed. Perhaps men who'd grown up in the late Victorian era learned it was impolite to smile for cameras. Perhaps being un-athletic and a bit too bookish made him lack self-assurance. Or, other reasons…perhaps his career after the war.

Likely, it was this last more than anything else.

Yet his work was nothing short of remarkable.

Ridley was the first to implant an artificial lens into the eye after cataract extraction, in 1949. The magnitude of this idea at the time cannot be exaggerated. It might have been comparable to the idea that an artificial heart was possible, but goes beyond a comparison such as this because the scientists who developed organ transplants

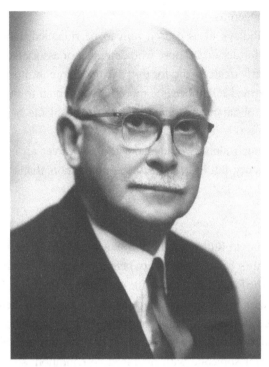

Harold Ridley.
Courtesy of the Estate of David Apple, M.D.

did so out of necessity and desperation – their patients would die unless they got a new heart or kidney or liver. Ridley's innovation was different, and courageous, because he made it at a time when most ophthalmologists thought they had already perfected cataract surgery. They believed this despite the fact that after surgery their patients no longer had a lens, a condition termed *aphakia,* and therefore needed very thick "coke bottle" glasses to focus light onto the retina and see a clear image. The surgery also required a week-long hospital stay. Still, ophthalmologists, as a group, congratulated themselves for having mastered the operation; and for someone like Ridley to challenge the status quo, to consider putting something *foreign* into the eye, like a lens implant, was ludicrous, heretical, and worse – dangerous.

Thus Ridley's ideas caused him to be ridiculed, ignored, and ostracized for decades. Those who defended or associated with him were similarly treated. And for thirty years, before intraocular lenses (usually termed IOLs) became more fully accepted in the 1980s, a generation of cataract patients were deprived of the best cure for aphakia.

This much alone would make Ridley's career an entertaining underdog story. But Ridley's story was much more than that.

In 1906, Harold Ridley was born into a world of Victorian gentility, when Britain's Empire was at its height. His father, Nicholas, had served in the Royal Navy, but while stationed in China he developed hemorrhages in his joints and was diagnosed with hemophilia. Discharged from the military, he decided to go to medical school. He'd wanted to be a general surgeon, but this was considered too strenuous for someone with his bleeding condition, so instead he became an ophthalmologist.

Harold was a studious boy who attended excellent prep schools, then Cambridge. He seems likely to have been the type of incorruptible young man that some parents are lucky to have – the kind that never gets into trouble and always earns straight As. He decided to follow his father into medicine, and subsequently, like his father, chose to become an ophthalmologist, securing a training spot at Moorfields Eye Hospital in London, the preeminent eye hospital in the world. Ridley was right where an up-and-coming physician should be. In a macabre sort of way, it didn't hurt that he was at the young end of the "lost generation" – the cohort of British men whose numbers had been decimated by World War I, a war which Ridley had been too young to fight in. Because of this demographic anomaly, ophthalmology, like many other professions at this time in England, experienced a dearth of practitioners. So young doctors expected to rise rapidly, and Ridley was flattered when Sir Stewart Duke-Elder, the most respected ophthalmologist in Britain, and probably the world, wrote him a wonderful letter of recommendation to be accepted as a consultant (what the British call their senior doctors or attendings) at Moorfields. Best of all, he was learning cataract surgery from England's finest. He liked the surgery, and found he was quite skilled at it.

For centuries, the treatment for cataract was a barbaric procedure called *couching,* in which a long needle was stabbed through the front of the eye and into the cataract in an attempt to dislodge it and push it into the back of the eye where it would sink into the vitreous – the thick gel that fills the eye's center. Not surprisingly, the technique was fraught with complications, most commonly infection and hemorrhage. Amazingly, it is still performed in some remote parts of the world today.

The technique Ridley learned in the mid-1930s was called *intracapsular* cataract extraction. A large, semicircular incision would be made around the rim of the cornea, through which one could use forceps to grasp the entire cataract and extract it. The eye was then sewn up with ten or twelve stitches. This was certainly a major improvement over couching, but there was a big drawback. Once the cataractous lens was gone, there was nothing left to focus the light rays onto the retina. Without a lens, a patient's vision is very blurry – in some cases, even blurrier than before the surgery.

In 1938, Ridley joined the staff at Moorfields Hospital as a full consultant at the relatively young age of 32. Then, one seemingly innocuous incident occurred that would have far-reaching implications for his career.

He made an enemy.

He didn't mean for it to happen, and later wished he'd handled it differently, but it was too late. His enemy was the most influential ophthalmologist in the world, Sir Stewart Duke-Elder, the same doctor who'd written him a letter of recommendation. The man was a legend. His fame primarily derived from authoring voluminous textbooks which became the canon of the field, required reading for a generation of ophthalmologists in the mid-twentieth century. After treating Prime Minister Ramsey MacDonald in 1932 for glaucoma, he was knighted. He was a high-browed Scotsman with a sharply angled nose, and a direct stare that could be very intimidating.

The problem began when Ridley, as an idealistic new consultant, saw room for improvement in the training program at Moorfields, which he believed had slipped in recent years. He wrote:

> Obviously something had to be done to put the hospital back to where it used to be before World War I – to restore it to be once more the ophthalmic center of excellence…There was to be a proper training program based on teaching good young men and not simply exploiting them to see far too many patients each day.

Ridley decided to shake things up. One of his first duties as a new consultant was to arrange staffing. Every consultant was responsible for supervising the eye clinic on his assigned day. This requirement had not been strictly enforced for the senior consultants, and certainly not for luminaries like Sir Duke-Elder, who sent younger associates to serve as substitutes. Ridley began enforcing this oft-ignored rule, and he also insisted that *all* consultants should perform surgery at the hospital, to share the workload and help train younger ophthalmologists. To this point, Duke-Elder had often sent proxy surgeons to fulfill his surgical obligations. These policies led to a serious row with Duke-Elder. It is possible that Duke-Elder strongly disliked performing surgery, a fact Ridley may not have known at the time. Perhaps Ridley's actions challenged Duke-Elder's entrenched seniority – we don't know all the details and neither man ever spoke publicly about it; but, we can surmise that Duke-Elder took great offense at Ridley's changes, for he began to treat Ridley as an adversary.

There was no way for Ridley to know, at the time, that becoming Duke-Elder's enemy would have a disastrous effect on his career.

He felt the first impact of this in 1941. World War II was on, and he was commissioned a Major in the Royal Army Medical Corps. Not surprisingly, Duke-Elder was the top ranking ophthalmologist in the Army, and hence had the power to station Britain's eye surgeons anywhere in the world. He sent Ridley to Ghana, in West Africa. It was an insulting assignment.

Ridley wrote, "This distressed me, for West Africa was not likely to be a fighting area where my surgical experience would be of value." In light of the high incidence of eye injuries during the war, there is no doubt his surgical expertise would have been better utilized as a frontline combat surgeon.

With time on his hands, Ridley dedicated himself to the study of onchocerciasis in northern Ghana, and published the first landmark study of the blinding parasitic disease that would become known as "river blindness." Victims of "river blindness" were infected with a roundworm called *Onchocerca volvulus*, which was transmitted by the bite of the black fly, an insect that bred in rivers and fast-moving streams. When the worms died, they triggered a severe host immune reaction; Ridley was the first to systematically document how the resulting inflammation damaged ocular tissues like the retina.

After a year and a half in Ghana, Ridley was transferred to India, and from there to Burma, where he was on the scene to examine released prisoners of war, many of whom had gone blind from malnourishment in Japanese labor camps. Ridley described the condition, which he termed, "nutritional amblyopia," and highlighted the visual impact of vitamin A deficiency.

> *I treated over 200 released allied prisoners of war in Rangoon and Singapore who suffered from nutritional amblyopia while Japanese prisoners of war. Many of the prisoners had worked on the Burma Railway. Starved and ill-treated, they had developed sudden central scotoma, relieved by good diet if available. Some developed optic atrophy, some of whom made a partial recovery within six weeks of release. However, the advanced cases, though given a vitamin-rich diet, were irreversible.*

Despite these accomplishments, Ridley no doubt still would have preferred to use his surgical skills to treat combat injuries. A few years earlier, in 1940, before going overseas to Africa, he'd treated RAF pilots during the Battle of Britain when he'd been working near Tangmere. The injuries had been horrific. There was one patient whom he couldn't forget, possibly because of his peculiar nickname, "Mouse," but also because his wounds were among the worst he'd ever seen. Dozens of tiny shards of plexiglass from his canopy had perforated Flight Lieutenant "Mouse" Cleaver's eyes. He had traumatic cataracts, was completely blind in his right eye, and almost blind in his left.

Mouse had been of a stoic sort. Ridley could tell that well enough by the dignified way he held his head, and the way he looked at a person who was speaking, even though he couldn't see and his injured eyes could make people gasp at their first sight of him. He also cared about his comrades. When his friend, a pilot named Jack Riddle, came to visit him in the hospital, the first thing Mouse said was, "Jack, tell them all to wear their goggles."

Ridley was fascinated by Mouse's injuries. To his surprise, the plexiglass foreign bodies in his eyes did not cause immediate infection, as any other foreign material would be expected to. In fact, there was not even any inflammation. Eye injuries from hot shrapnel, which he'd thought might be sterile, still caused infection and inflammation. So did lead bullet fragments. But apparently, not plexiglass. Ridley saw Mouse multiple times, confirming that the plexiglass always remained inert, well-tolerated by the eye. He later wrote, "…unless a sharp edge of the plastic material rests in contact with a sensitive and mobile portion of the eye, the tissue reaction is insignificant." At the time, he did not realize the extent to which meeting Mouse Cleaver would alter the course of his life.

When the war ended, Ridley returned to Moorfields and resumed practicing ophthalmology. Despite his skill at removing cataracts, it always bothered Ridley that, after the operation, the aphakic, lens-less patients still couldn't see very well, even *with* their thick "soda-pop" glasses, so-called because their shape resembled the glass at the bottom of a soda bottle. The view through these glasses was extremely distorted in the periphery; in effect, the patient could only hope for a small window of clear vision straight ahead. He believed, "extraction alone is but half the cure for cataract."

One day in 1948, a medical student named Stephen Perry was watching him operate. Perry was energetic and curious. He watched Ridley remove a cataract and commented, "Mr. Ridley," (consultants were called "Mr." at the time), "it's a pity you can't replace the cataract with a clear lens."

It was a naïve comment. Perry didn't know that there was no way to replace the lens. But the words flipped a switch in Ridley's mind. Remembering Mouse Cleaver's injuries, and the plastic plexiglass that had remained inert in his eyes, he suddenly wondered whether it might be possible to make an artificial lens of the same material and insert it into the eye.

This was a revolutionary idea. To that point, all surgical maneuvers in ophthalmology had been designed to *remove* things from the eye. Never before had anyone intentionally *put* something in the eye and left it there. Ridley felt certain it was possible, but understood that what he intended to try would be very controversial, and secrecy would be important. He quietly contacted John Pike, a scientist he knew at Raynor & Keeler, Ltd., a prominent British optical company. The two men met in Ridley's car, parked outside a public park. Of this meeting, he wrote,

> *While seated in the car, I explained the project and invited John Pike to join in a new and exciting venture and he enthusiastically agreed. Within perhaps half an hour, the cure of cataracts was established. We agreed to use an implant made of plastic, chemically sterilized and situated in the posterior chamber, where God had placed the human lens. John Pike was to calculate the necessary optical values required and he would also ask his friend…to produce some real high quality acrylic.*

With Ridley's input, Raynor & Keeler manufactured the first artificial intraocular lens (IOL). It was biconvex, like the natural lens, with an equatorial ridge that could be used to grasp and handle it using surgical instruments.

Ridley scheduled the first patient who would ever receive an intraocular lens implant for surgery on November 29, 1949, at St. Thomas Hospital, which was located across the Thames from the Houses of Parliament. The operation was a secret, with only a few trusted staff present. After removing the cataract, he inserted the IOL as he had planned; but, after he'd done it, he suddenly wasn't sure that it would stay in place. He made a difficult decision. He removed the IOL and closed the eye. He thought it might be better to insert it again in a subsequent surgery, after the postoperative inflammation had diminished. This second surgery was successfully performed on February 8, 1950.

Of the first two patients who volunteered for the surgery, Ridley wrote,

> We must not fail to honor two brave Londoners, who, though well aware of the dangers, risked the loss of an eye so that our future patients might benefit. To them ophthalmology owes a great debt; for all of us involved in the history of intraocular implants they are the true pioneers.

Ridley soon performed ten such operations. They were anatomically successful – the lenses were inserted into the eyes and well-tolerated. After the first two cases he quickly learned that the power of the IOL had to be adjusted, because the refractive power of the lens in the aqueous fluid of the eye was much different from its power in the open air, an assumption which had not been accounted for. The inserted IOLs were supported by the lens capsule, which had been purposely left behind, but even so, the weight of these early lenses made them prone to dislocate toward the bottom of the eye. This would prove to be a major complication of the surgery, and some of the dislocated IOLs had to be removed.

Ridley did not intend to publish and share the results of his surgeries for up to two years, giving him time to build a large series of patients and make a strong case for the use of IOLs. However, as fate would have it, one patient's innocent mistake thwarted this plan, and set in motion a series of unpleasant events that had unfortunate results for him, and in fact, for the world.

One of Ridley's patients wanted to schedule a follow-up appointment with him. He looked in the phone book and dialed the number of Frederick Ridley, another ophthalmologist in London. The patient went to the appointment, was examined by the other Mr. Ridley, and the secret was out.

Ridley was compelled to accelerate the unveiling of his work. He scrambled to finish the articles he was working on and sent them out. Already, the word had spread like wildfire. He was in the spotlight.

The response was not good.

Many of Ridley's peers considered the idea of an artificial lens to be reckless malpractice. Critics excoriated him for his complications, which included corneal edema, glaucoma, and IOL dislocation. They raised questions about theoretical complications, such as sympathetic ophthalmia, a severe autoimmune reaction that affects the fellow eye, and even malignancy. Ridley became distressed over the real possibility that he might be sued, or lose his hospital privileges.

His most public rejection occurred in the most prominent of forums, the Oxford Ophthalmological Congress in July 1951, one of the most important meetings in the field at the time. His presentation was carefully prepared, including slides, films, and even two of his patients who had regained vision of 20/20 and 20/15 in their operated eyes, appearing in person. He would offer to let the other ophthalmologists examine the patients.

The response to his presentation was not at all what he expected. In later years, he wrote down these memories of the conference:

In spite of my request for favorable timing, the Hon. Secretary

*of the Oxford Congress arranged presentation of this paper just
after the lunch break, when some members had not returned to
the lecture hall. Two delighted patients had traveled to Oxford
in my car, one refusing to agree that the time on the clock was 5
minutes to the hour, insisting rightly, without glasses, that it was
3 minutes to the hour. These patients, one of whose result was
perfect...aroused interest and disbelief. Sir Stewart Duke-Elder
and others repeatedly refused even to look at my demonstration
patients...There were a few further trifling comments and then
suddenly the Deputy Master foreclosed the discussion, an action
for which he apologized later in the day.*

Perplexed by the unequivocally negative reception of his work,
Ridley began to suspect that his old nemesis, Sir Duke-Elder, had
poisoned many of ophthalmology's elite against his new idea. On
other occasions, Ridley recalled the meeting this way:

*There was, however, one powerful opponent, a British
ophthalmologist justly famous for his splendid writings rather
than for treatment of patients. He firmly refused repeated
requests to look at the patients, so confirming his hostility even
at that very early stage.*

*When the presentation of the paper ended there was a little more
applause than usual and a few questions. In general there was
surprisingly little comment...At later meetings some wounding
comments were made in many countries.*

But such measured comments belie the viciousness with which
his ideas were met by the ophthalmology establishment. Comments
from his peers included:

"Dr. Ridley, why don't you...GO HOME."

"Would you have one of THESE THINGS put in your son's eye?"

*"As long as I remain in charge of this department no implant will ever
be done."*

"This operation should never be done."

"It offends the first principle of ophthalmic surgery…"

At a meeting of the American Academy of Ophthalmology in Chicago in 1952, Dr. Derrik Vail, the editor-in-chief of the *American Journal of Ophthalmology* and a close friend of Duke-Elder's, publicly stated:

> In spite of Mr. Ridley's remarkably successful run of cases reported here, the operation is one of considerable recklessness. Its hazards far exceed the little that is gained in the way of ocular comfort to the patient and the questionable advantage of binocular vision obtained at such an obvious risk.
>
> Until further work is done and more time has elapsed…I do not want such an operation performed on myself nor can I advise it for my patients, willing as they might be to undergo the additional hazards of which they can have no true conception.

For the next twenty years, Ridley's time at Moorfields was very difficult. He encountered hostility to his ideas, and those who sided with him earned the scorn of Duke-Elder and other well-established ophthalmologists. Ridley once recalled that one of his friends "received a personal warning from Duke-Elder against cooperating with me – a threat that if he continued to support me he would never get a consultant post."

Although he continued working and operating, Ridley sank into depression. He was not outspoken and did not fight back against his critics. One of the reasons for this was his fear of facing allegations of malpractice and attracting lawsuits. There *were* serious complications that needed to be improved and addressed in addition to IOL dislocation, such as reliably predicting the proper IOL power for individual patients and handling opacification of the lens capsule, a common occurrence that often required another surgery. But these problems were solvable, and the opposition to Ridley's work only delayed the necessary research and proper clinical trials needed to improve techniques of IOL implantation for decades. Ridley's biographer, Dr. David Apple, wrote of this time:

> Many ophthalmologists and their patients experienced unfavorable results during the many years of often chaotic experimentation and defective IOL design and manufacture prior to the current re-establishment of Ridley's principles. Some lenses between the mid-1950s and the mid-1980s were of such poor quality that it was often sarcastically joked that they would have made better IUDs than IOLs.

In 1971, Ridley formally retired from Moorfields. In his own words, he was being "put out to pasture."

We know now that intraocular lenses have restored the sight of millions around the world, but it was not until well after Ridley retired that the proponents of IOLs began to make serious inroads against the opposition. Slowly, more and more surgeons around the world began to try and adopt IOLs. In 1980, more than thirty years after Ridley's first groundbreaking surgery, the American FDA held a hearing on the safety profile of IOLs. Even then, the outcome was in serious doubt. In the end, some say the testimony of Robert Young, well-known as "America's Doctor" for his television role as Marcus Welby, M.D., was critical to the decision to uphold the use of IOLs. Having had the operation in both eyes, Young said, "Let me tell you, IOLs saved my career and should be made available to all Americans."

It is unfortunate that the decades of opposition likely contributed to Ridley's years of depression. Knowing this, it isn't surprising that he looks grim in most photos. Yet there are also accounts of Ridley's warmth and sense of humor, which provide a more rounded view of him. A student who asked him for advice about going into ophthalmology wrote of him,

> I recall him as a slight man with a round pink face and a small moustache. He wore a binocular magnifier strapped to his forehead, which he hinged upwards when not in use. This gave

him a somewhat jaunty appearance as he spoke. He was direct and to the point and I suspected a streak of humour was never very far away. "Yes, there is no reason why you should not take up ophthalmology. No, you don't have to be particularly bright. You will never go hungry, although you might occasionally go a little thirsty..."

The same person became a resident and wrote this about learning surgery from Ridley:

Harold's method of teaching was immensely reassuring to the beginner. He would assist at one's side for the first few moments of the operation and then, when the serious stuff had to be done, he would move over, to take up a position under the tall windows above his head, which overlooked Lambeth Palace Road. Here he would proceed to examine his fingernails with the most scrupulous attention, apparently so completely confident of the successful outcome of the operation that his closer presence was deemed entirely unnecessary...Later, sometimes much later, when the tension had gone, he might offer some criticism – "Rather small flap, Walker" – and get into his car.

In 1989 and 1990, Ridley himself underwent cataract extraction and IOL implantation and attained 20/20 vision in each eye. By this time, IOLs had become the standard of care. He had been vindicated. In his estimation, resistance to his ideas "delayed the cure of aphakia for twenty-five years so that an entire generation of cataract patients needlessly suffered aphakia."

Ridley was fortunate to live to see his efforts recognized. He received many honors, the most meaningful of which was being knighted by Queen Elizabeth II on February 9, 2000, at the age of 93. Two stamps honoring him were issued by the British Postal Service in 2003. He never patented his IOL and never earned a cent from it. He believed his invention belonged to humankind.

Ridley died in Salisbury, England on May 25, 2001.

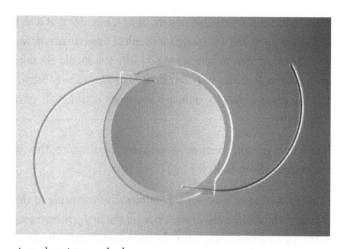

A modern intraocular lens.
© 2002 American Academy of Ophthalmology.

It is estimated that about eight million cataract surgeries with IOL implantation are performed annually around the world. Today, IOLs are so advanced that they can be folded to fit through a 1.8 mm incision and then open up inside the eye as they are guided into position. Multifocal IOLs permit patients to see both near and far. Refractive IOLs are implanted into the healthy eyes of young people who have never had cataract surgery as an alternative to refractive surgery.

The treatment for cataract did not progress one iota for centuries. In the last thirty years, it has advanced at warp speed. We owe a debt to Sir Harold Ridley, whose inspiration came from examining a pilot whose eyes had been pierced by shards of plexiglass, and whose quiet dignity and perseverance ultimately triumphed over his detractors and depression.

In 1987, the traumatic cataract in Flight Lieutenant Mouse Cleaver's left eye was removed. He received an intraocular lens, and regained sight in that eye.

Chapter Three | *"The delicious sensation of that*
ultrasonic probe against my teeth..."

CHARLES KELMAN AND PHACOEMULSIFICATION

When an ophthalmology resident learns how to do cataract surgery for the first time, he or she is introduced to an instrument and technique that has no similarity to anything he has seen in other medical specialties. No previously learned surgical skills can be applied here. Nor does a childhood history of playing lots of video games help, either. The technique, invented by Charles Kelman, M.D., is called *phacoemulsification*.

"Phaco" (Greek for "lens") has become synonymous with cataract extraction because it is the most efficient way of removing cataracts. When Harold Ridley removed a cataract, he made a large, semicircular incision around the cornea – it *had* to be big so that the whole cataract could be extracted in one piece. Then, ten to twelve sutures were required to close the wound. Ridley's patients would be immobilized in the hospital for a week, and recover at home over an additional 6-8 weeks.

Charles Kelman wanted to find a better way to remove cataracts, through small incisions, with less recovery time. And he succeeded: today our incisions are as small as 1.8 millimeters wide, and don't even have to be sutured at all. Patients see well and are able to go home the same day.

Of course, when ophthalmology residents are learning this technique, most couldn't care less who invented it, or how great the story of its invention was. Their sole objective is to become competent as quickly as possible so that fewer patients may suffer from their inexperience.

The phacoemulsification probe has a tip that vibrates rapidly, but only a miniscule amount, emitting ultrasonic energy to emulsify a cataract. When the novice resident first sits down next to the patient's head in the operating room, all he sees is an exposed eyeball, lids spread apart with a metal speculum. Everything else is covered up by a blue drape. Suddenly one realizes there are a whole lot of controls. First, there's the phaco machine, which is about as tall as a half-sized refrigerator, on wheels. The machine has a multitude of settings: power, vacuum, aspiration, bottle height, pulse, polish, vitrectomy, and others. There's a foot pedal for each foot, one to control the machine and one to focus the operating microscope. Getting used to the sensitivity of the pedals takes time. Press down just a little and all you get is fluid flowing out the phaco tip. A little more pressure and the tip emits energy to break up the cataract. Press down still more and it begins sucking – to evacuate the lens pieces. Both hands, both feet, are engaged, active. It takes coordination, a little like driving stick while parallel parking on a downhill slope.

Despite all this, I was pretty confident going into my first phaco case, during my second year of residency. I'd gotten it into my head that cataract surgery should be a piece of cake. Maybe it's because I'd watched many attendings do it with ease. They were *fast*, sometimes doing up to sixteen cases a day. Maybe it's because the patients' expectations were very high, since their friends and relatives had already had smooth operations. They expected to see very well the next day and have perfect distance vision. There seemed to be a general assumption that cataract surgery should take ten minutes, fifteen at most – how hard could it be?

Plenty hard.

Under the microscope, all my movements looked grotesquely exaggerated. I had no awareness that my hand was moving, but under magnification, there was a tiny tremor that was embarrassingly obvious to me and my attending. When the patient shifted a little it was like watching an earthquake. I started the case and attempted to use a needle with a bent tip to score a hole in the front of the thin, delicate lens capsule. I'd seen it done dozens of times. I'd practiced it on model eyes. But this time, with a live patient, I found that I couldn't even *see* the capsule itself.

I focused up, raising the microscope. I focused down, lowering it. *The capsule's invisible!*

Of course it is, I realized, *it's supposed to be transparent.*

How could I operate on something I couldn't see?

I couldn't, so I just sat there, frozen, for seconds that seemed like hours. My attending cleared his throat; he was wondering what I was waiting for, so I began to probe around with the needle, mimicking the movements I'd seen attendings perform, sweating the whole time.

Finally, after my attending had helped me complete the hole in the lens capsule, I got to the part where I could start to emulsify the cataract. *Great, let 'er rip,* I figured. But this part of the procedure was no easier. There wasn't much room to move in the front of the eye. I prayed I wouldn't injure the back of the cornea or chew up the iris. I believed I was getting at the lens when in fact I was carving up nothing – I was still way above it.

Afterwards, I left the operating room, shaking my head, and thinking, *It's harder than I thought. OK, much harder. Still, it has to get easier, right?*

But my first case had taken me forty-five minutes. How could I ever do it in ten?

What really concerned me was that I couldn't see the capsule and didn't have a good sense of depth under the microscope. A thought flashed in my head – *What if I don't have stereovision?*

I ran to the pediatric department and checked out the 3-D vision tests they do on kids. *Whew.* I still saw the monkeys jumping off the page.

I did more cases. With each one, I improved, performing at least one aspect of the surgery with more grace. I got better at seeing the capsule. Better at controlling the phaco tip. Better at judging how deep to carve the lens.

After about ten or fifteen cases, things started really clicking. I suddenly saw everything, every layer, every groove I was making. The patient would move and my foot would adjust the scope without my thinking about it. I got my time down to fifteen minutes. Patients, as expected, were doing well and seeing great the next day. I was becoming a skilled cataract surgeon.

When I was able to stop worrying about every movement I made during surgery, I began to realize what an ingenious invention this phacoemulsifier was, the instrument that made the experience so easy for the doctor and the patient. It was a true marvel. Unique, in that it hadn't evolved from another surgical instrument; it wasn't a newfangled scalpel or suction device, modified to fit in the eye. No, it was completely different from anything else used in surgery. A surgery that used to take over an hour, ten stitches, and a week in the hospital, now took a fraction of the time, with the added benefit of seeing smiling patients the next day.

After one case, near the end of my residency, I was chatting with an older attending who'd trained in the 1970's. He was telling me about the *old days*. He chuckled when he remembered admitting patients to the hospital *before* their cataract surgery, and rounding on them for a week. "They were poor old saps," he remembered, "spending days lying on their backs, frozen, heads locked in place with sandbags on either side. How far we've come," he mused, shaking his head.

"Who invented this machine?" I asked.

"Charley Kelman," he said.

"One guy?"

"Yes, one guy, but he was really interesting," the doctor said, smiling knowingly.

"Interesting?"

"He was...a performer," he said. "He trained here at Wills, too, you know. Read up on him, you'll see what I mean."

———

New York City, 1965

Charley Kelman was miserable.

And tired.

He opened the door to the dentist's office, entering a drab reception room with a linoleum floor and circular brown water stains dotting the drop-down ceiling panels. The chairs didn't match, some faded wood, others plastic. A couple of cheaply framed Norman Rockwell prints adorned the plain gray walls.

Kelman checked in and sat down. A black and white TV droned in the corner, the image flickering spasmodically. An old lady was hunched over in a corner, fiddling with her dentures and, at intervals, making a strange sucking sound.

The whole scene mirrored the way Kelman felt.

He rubbed his chin, scratched at the stubble. He hadn't shaved for four days. This morning, looking in the mirror, he'd stared at his disheveled hair; he was beginning to look like one of the hippies loitering around Columbia University.

But Kelman was no hippie. He was a doctor, an ophthalmologist. A surgeon. He was building his practice in Manhattan, and it was growing. He had a wife and three kids. He should be happy, but he wasn't. And his hair was way too long.

Everything he'd worked for over the previous two years had come to nothing. All because of an obsession with one *idea,* one hare-brained idea that wouldn't go away. He was sure he could invent a better way to remove cataracts through a small incision. But he'd failed, and his obsession was keeping him from his wife and kids. His heart felt as cold as the vat of liquid nitrogen he'd just stored in his lab.

What had gone wrong? With him? His idea? His life?

He'd been a happy-go-lucky kid, who wanted to be a musician, a saxman, when he grew up. *That* had made him happy, his dream of becoming a star. And he was good, too. Even now, the memory of the song he'd recorded and gotten on the radio made him smile – *Telephone Numbers* by Kerry Adams – a name he'd made up because he was worried that his attendings would disapprove.

Maybe I *should* have been a musician, he mused.

But then, he remembered why he'd become a doctor.

His father's advice echoed in his head: "Son, it's your life. You can do with it whatever you like. You can be a songwriter, a singer, a saxophone player, or any other kind of bum you want. But first, you'll be a doctor." His father always dispensed advice empathetically, but he was also firm. He left no doubt about what he expected Charley to do. Yes, his son had a talent for music, but in his opinion, being a doctor, first and foremost, was the only choice.

So Kelman *had* become a doctor. He'd become an ophthalmologist. But now he knew he'd never be content just being an ordinary doctor; he was happy only when performing in front of others. He admitted to himself that the thing he loved most of all was being the center of attention. It was intoxicating. No matter what, he still wanted to be a star.

The insatiable drive to *be* someone, to *do* something really great was what had gotten him into this mess, so that now, sitting in a dentist's office, he was staring failure in the face.

He'd thought he could make a name for himself in ophthalmology, maybe invent something important – perhaps that would be his way of becoming famous. He hated being anonymous, sitting in the back row of the big ophthalmology meetings, watching the big shots of the field stride across the stage, joking with each other on a first name basis from behind the podium. *He* wanted to be at the podium. He wanted *his* name to be remembered, in reference to an operation he'd developed, a surgical instrument he'd invented, something that had lasting merit in the field of medicine. If he was going to be a doctor, he'd better be a famous one.

He took in the dentist's outdated magazines, scattered across the coffee table in front of him. A *magazine*...he remembered...it had all started with the cover of *Look* magazine. There'd been a surgeon on the cover one day, wearing a mask in an operating room. Dr. Irving S. Cooper, neurosurgeon. The article on Dr. Cooper explained how he'd developed a freezing probe, which he used to freeze parts of the brain, to cure Parkinson's disease. The man actually kept patients awake in the OR, so their hands would keep trembling. He used X-rays to determine exactly where in the brain he wanted his probe to be positioned, and then he started freezing. Then, right before his eyes, the tremors would stop, the hands would go still, and Dr. Cooper would stop freezing.

The freezing probe had given Kelman a bright idea. Why couldn't this freezing treatment be used to treat retinal tears? Up to that point, retinal tears had been treated with a *hot* probe. The probe was placed on the sclera, over the area of the tear, and the heat made a scar that would adhere the retina to the eye wall. This was designed to prevent the tear from causing a retinal detachment. Problem was, the heat weakened and thinned the sclera itself, so much so that sometimes it actually went *through* the eye wall, a disastrous result.

What if a freezing treatment could make the scar, but not perforate the sclera?

Kelman felt sure a cold probe would work. He went to Dr. Cooper's office and introduced himself. The neurosurgeon agreed to let him work in his lab, and Kelman started experimenting.

His first experiments were on cats. Looking inside the eye as he activated the probe, he saw the retina get white as the ice ball formed. Then, it thawed and looked normal again. Later, a perfect, adherent scar developed.

It worked.

Next Kelman wondered – what would freezing do to other parts of the eye? He tried a cat's lens and the probe froze to it, bonding with it until it thawed. *That's it!* he realized. *This could be a great way to remove cataracts.*

Of course, cataract surgery at the time was already considered quite refined, successful in ninety percent of cases. But Kelman knew the surgery and the patient's recovery were not easy. After cutting a large incision, the surgeon would reach through the pupil and grasp the lens with forceps. Then he would pull the lens out, rupturing all the tiny supporting *zonules* that normally held it in place.

This would usually go smoothly, except when the hold on the lens was slippery, or loose, and the surgeon's grasp on the cataract might slip. Even worse, the lens capsule might tear, with cataract pieces falling into the back of the eye where they could cause severe inflammation or retinal problems. Kelman's freezing probe could eliminate these problems by solidly bonding to the cataract, eliminating the risk of capsule rupture or losing hold of the lens. He started trying it on patients, and it worked each time. He knew this would also be a better way to handle cataracts in children, and traumatic cataracts, too.

Kelman's goal was innocent enough – recognition, respect, and possibly fame, but all for the right intentions. His invention, or adaptation, was all for the good, to help others. If they called it the *Kelman procedure,* so be it.

He was on cloud nine.

But, when he submitted his article about freezing the retina to *Ophthalmology*, the premier scientific journal in the field, it was rejected. Then, he got another surprise. Dr. Cooper called him and told him one of his colleagues, a retinal surgeon from Eastern University, had contacted him to discuss collaborating on a project to study freezing of the retina. Cooper intended to do it. "Eastern has the facilities, the prestige, the money," he told Kelman. "Continue with the cataract investigation. Don't try to hog it all."

Kelman was convinced that whoever this retinal person was, he had reviewed his article, rejected it, and stolen his idea. And when he applied to present his work at the meeting of the American Academy of Ophthalmology, the most prestigious meeting of its kind in the country, he was told the doctors from Eastern had already been awarded the spot on the program for it.

Though understandably furious, Kelman was undeterred. He still had the idea of freezing the lens. He was sure he'd make his mark using the freezing probe on cataracts.

Until he read a report by Dr. Theodorus Krawicz from Poland. He'd just done the same exact thing – frozen a lens and extracted it from the eye. He'd published first. Here, again, Kelman was too late. It was little solace when the Academy let him present his cataract research at the meeting, for after he'd spoken, several in the audience laughed. It was commented that he had used a sixty thousand dollar machine to do the job the rest of them could do with a two dollar forceps.

Now, sitting in the dentist's office, Kelman cringed over these memories.

A nurse appeared at the reception door.

"Charles Kelman," she said, reading his name.

Kelman pulled himself up and followed her into the dental suite, a little surprised to find the patient chair to be shiny and new. The lamp hanging from the ceiling was stainless steel, the dental instruments perfectly arranged on a tray. This sparkling interior bore little resemblance to the near squalor of the outer office.

Guess he's put all his money into the equipment, he thought.

Settling into the chair, Kelman stared at the posters from national parks which had been used to decorate the ceiling. Yosemite Valley. The Grand Canyon. He liked them. He thought about all the patients with cataracts who wouldn't be able to enjoy the view like he could. But he had lost faith that he would ever be able to do what he'd wanted to do for them – make cataract surgery better, faster, and less burdensome.

Six more weeks before the grant is up, he recalled.

The three-year, $299,000 grant from the Hartford Foundation. How he'd celebrated when he'd been awarded the money three years ago, promising to deliver on small incision cataract surgery. He didn't have concrete ideas at the time, but he'd won the grant using charm and showmanship, and at that time he figured it was only a little while before he found the answer.

Still working on cats' eyes, one whole year went into developing a small rubber net. But the net was too big, it broke too often and caused too much damage inside the eye. He next tried a series of high speed drills for pulverizing the lens. For some reason, although the cataract would get broken up, the cats' corneas always came out opaque, white and traumatized, even though the cornea hadn't been touched. It took another year for him to realize the drill was throwing off thousands of tiny lens fragments which would crash into the backside of the cornea, where the endothelial cells, responsible for keeping the cornea clear by continually dehydrating it, were being irreversibly destroyed. Finally, he'd tried different chemicals to dissolve the cataract, but nothing worked. After spending just about $300,000, he had nothing to show for it, and he was going to have to report it to the Foundation. He'd be the laughingstock of ophthalmology.

Kelman was at the very bottom of a downward spiral. He was a failed inventor who'd wasted years of his life. He loved his family, but couldn't deny that his work had taken its toll on them, too. In the midst of all this, he wondered why he couldn't just be satisfied being a regular eye doctor. The money was fine. What was wrong with a nice house in the suburbs, a country club membership, and a couple good vacations each year? Why wasn't that enough?

The door swung open. A handsome man in his forties sauntered in.

"Hi Dr. Kelman, I'm Larry Kuhn," the dentist said with a ready smile.

Kelman returned the greeting half-heartedly. The dentist washed his hands. Kelman was surprised he was going to do the cleaning himself, rather than a hygienist.

"Let's see what we have," Kuhn said as he sat down beside his patient. Kelman opened his mouth. He was almost too embarrassed to do it – his teeth were yellow from smoking countless cigarettes. Brushing was a habit he seldom made time for. Kuhn poked around with a mirror and probe, muttering, "Um hm. Um hmmm."

At least I'm not a dentist, Kelman thought, *digging around in people's mouths all day.* The notion both disgusted and consoled him at the same time.

Kuhn reached over to the instrument stand and retrieved a slender silver instrument. He depressed a pedal and it emitted a high-pitched hum. There was a fine mist coming from the end, but the tip wasn't moving.

"Let's get to work," he said.

When the instrument touched Kelman's teeth, it presented the feeling of rapid vibration, and a tingling sensation that was completely foreign – it wasn't painful, but the surprise made him pull back his head and push the dentist's hand away, startling him.

"What is that?" Kelman said.

Kuhn regained his composure. "This? Ah, it's my new baby. It's an ultrasonic probe. Vibrates twenty-five thousand times a second. That's how it can clean your teeth, picking off those particles of tartar, without you feeling it. It's a question of acceleration."

Kelman felt a strange elation begin to well up in his chest, the beginning of an idea forming in his head, and he knew it would be a good one: *this probe carving up a cataract...* he looked at the narrow tip... *through a tiny incision. This was it!*

He leapt out of the chair and hugged Kuhn, kissing him on both cheeks.

"What the hell's the matter with you?" Kuhn shouted, pushing Kelman away.

"Larry, you just saved my life!"

Kelman ran out of the office and jumped into his car, the dental bib still around his neck. He spun out of the parking lot.

Twenty minutes later he was back. With a jar in his hand, he marched back into Kuhn's exam room. Kuhn stared at him, not knowing whether to call the police.

"Wait a second, Larry. Just let me try something."

Kelman unscrewed the jar and took out a cataract, one that had been extracted from a patient earlier that day. When he applied the probe to the cataract, it made smooth grooves, without moving the lens itself, one of the main problems he'd encountered when using the drill. Because of its ludicrously high tip velocity, this ultrasonic probe emulsified the cataract without bouncing the lens around or throwing off a multitude of tiny lens pieces.

He knew it would work.

He was about to be famous.

———

Years later, in his autobiography, Kelman wrote about the moment at the dentist's office.

> *I knew it wouldn't be quite that easy, that the instrument would have to be modified, perhaps a hundred times, but I also knew that I had found, finally, in the eleventh hour, the road that would lead to small incision cataract surgery. I sat back and let*

Larry finish his work on me. I reveled in the delicious sensation
of that ultrasonic probe against my teeth.

Kelman's next move was to contact Cavitron, the company that made the dental instrument. Unfortunately, they weren't interested in making a machine for the eye.

But Kelman persisted, and he finally convinced Cavitron to produce a prototype. He worked around the clock. He designed a hole in the probe to permit suction, for removal of the emulsified lens particles. It took him forty-five minutes to emulsify a cat's lens; but, although the eyes looked good at the end of surgery, they were always inflamed or infected the next day. He couldn't figure out why, until he realized the probe was getting extremely hot, from friction, up to well over a hundred degrees – so hot that he was actually cooking the eyeball! So he designed a sleeve with a continuous infusion of cold saline around the probe tip to keep it cool. He called the procedure *Phacoemulsification and Aspiration.*

This was about the fortieth prototype he'd developed in his pursuit of a better way to evacuate the lens. Kelman later described how the phaco probe was different from the dozens of microdrills he'd tried.

At the end of two years, with most of my grant money spent, the solution to the problem of lens movement and denuding of the corneal endothelium had become more than a challenge: it was an obsession. I realized that to be successful, the technique had to ensure that the lens remained stationary in the chamber. Acceleration of the moving tip against the lens had to be high enough so that its standing inertia would not be overcome, high enough so that the lens could not back away, vibrate, or rotate with the tip. To illustrate this principle, imagine a sharp knife slowly pushing against a punching bag. The punching bag will move with the movement of the knife. If, however, the knife is quickly plunged against the bag, it will penetrate and the bag will not move.

Finally, with this probe – and for the first time – he was ready to try it on a human patient.

He wanted to find patients with cataracts in eyes that were already blind, or were so painful they were already slated to be *enucleated,* that is, removed. If the surgery did not succeed, he did not want to be damaging an eye that could otherwise see. He made sure the patients understood that this was an experimental procedure and that they would not regain sight from it, but that perhaps future patients would.

His first patient was John Martin, who had gone blind from glaucoma. His eye had become painful and was scheduled for enucleation. Like Harold Ridley before him, and with as much reason, Kelman was paranoid about secrecy. He wasn't going to have his discovery usurped this time. Only a few trusted staff were present. When the anesthesiologist asked what his new machine was, he kept his answers vague. He chose a time when other ophthalmologists were busy working in their offices and wouldn't be in the hospital. He opted for an operating room at the end of the hall, away from the others, all in an effort to reduce the chance that a colleague might pop his or her head in for a look.

The case started out well. He was grooving troughs in John Martin's cataract just like he'd practiced many times in a cat. Then, suddenly the dome of the cornea inverted and was sucked into the probe's tip.

Oh no!

Kelman took his foot off the pedal, but it was too late.

He knew this was a disaster. There was no doubt he'd traumatized the cornea and failed. This had never happened in the cat's eye.

How had it happened? He had no idea. By now his staff was sensing something was wrong. He decided to go on.

He started grooving the cataract again. And – *No!* – it happened again. The cornea got sucked into the tip and then the anterior chamber, the small space between the lens and the cornea, collapsed.

Distressed, Kelman forced himself to go on, gingerly, carefully.

To make things worse, the pupil began to constrict and he could no longer see the peripheral lens that was behind the iris.

Finally, completely exhausted, he stopped.

Later, he wrote about the results of this first case:

I looked at the eye. It was horrible. The cornea had deep white lines etched into it. The iris had been touched several times by the emulsifier and was ragged, chewed away…When I got up from the chair, I again looked at the clock. Four and a half hours, seventy-nine minutes of which were emulsification time. I had been sitting in one position so long I had cut off the circulation to my legs. I swayed as I stood, holding onto the table. My clothes and the operating gown were drenched. The anesthesiologist looked at me as if I were insane. I dragged myself to an adjacent, unused operating room where I stretched out on the table, telling myself that everything was going to be alright…

He stayed at John Martin's bedside all night. The next morning he examined the eye – it was full of pus.

That afternoon he enucleated the eye.

In the days that followed, Kelman was a haunted man, haunted by John Martin's eye, haunted by the years of work, haunted by the lost time with his wife and children, and the ridicule of his peers.

He pinpointed the problem. The probe was drawing up lens particles as intended, but – once the particles were fully sucked up and the probe tip was suddenly clear, anything and everything could be drawn to the tip – the suction was too high, so strong that the cornea itself had been sucked down into it.

He needed to find a way to control the flow through the tip, so that the suction would shut off when the tip was cleared of lens pieces.

He spent two years searching for the answer. Finally, he found a company that had developed an electronic flow meter that would be able to stop the machine when it sensed a sudden rise in suction. He updated his equipment and got ready to try again.

He found a new patient, named Anna, a seventy-year-old woman. The surgery took three hours. It was painstaking, difficult work. But there were no collapses like the first time. The day after the surgery, the eye was intact, and not infected. It had been a success. Kelman did four more operations over the next six months. Each time he got better at it. All the eyes healed well afterwards.

One day, Kelman operated on the right eye of Abe Levin, whose left eye had gone blind from macular degeneration. Levin's right eye was also almost sightless, where his cataract was so severe that it was impossible to view the macula. Kelman assumed the right macula was just as damaged as the left macula was.

The case went smoothly.

But a short time later, Kelman was informed that he was being investigated by the hospital's medical board. It had been reported that he was performing "experimental surgery" and that he had "blinded four people." If the charges were true, he would be expelled from the hospital, his reputation damaged for life.

How had they gotten wind of this? He'd kept everything secret.

When he looked for the patients' records he realized they were all gone, as was his private diary detailing the cases. *What was going on?* He couldn't have misplaced them. *Had they been stolen?*

Immediately he thought of the employee he'd recently caught embezzling from his practice. She'd been more than a little disgruntled, and probably now hated him. *She* must have taken the records...but he had no proof.

Kelman expected an inquisition. He had enemies on the hospital staff, men who didn't like his flamboyant style, or were perhaps jealous of him. He knew the majority of the members on the panel would be against him.

But he also knew that he had done nothing wrong, that all the patients had given fully informed consent; though, without his patient records, he couldn't prove anything. The day of the hearing came. He brought a well-dressed man to the meeting; the board assumed it was his lawyer.

The hospital panel began to ask pointed questions about all the complications he had had: corneal trauma, collapsing anterior chambers, iris damage, pupil constriction. It was obvious that they had read his diary. Then the final accusation was made, that all of the patients were blind after surgery.

Kelman got his chance to speak. He explained that he had only operated on eyes that were blind before surgery.

Did he have records proving this? they asked.

No, the records had disappeared.

The panel scoffed their disbelief.

Now Kelman nodded to his companion.

The well-dressed man, who up to this point had remained seated and inconspicuous, opened a brief case and began to read a typed letter.

> *Gentlemen, it is the surgeon's right and duty to perform what he considers to be the best procedure for his patient. That Dr. Kelman chose not to inform you of the type of operation he was doing is his right. He did what he and his patients thought best…Let me now address myself to the success or failure of Dr. Kelman's technique. Dr. Kelman has stated that until now, all the operations have been on eyes that had no ability to see. Two days ago, however, Dr. Kelman did, most definitely operate on a patient with useful vision: the first of many such patients who will benefit from his technique. I will now prove to you the success of the operation.*

The man put the paper down, closed the brief case, and removed his glasses. He put a patch around his head and pulled it down over his left eye. Suddenly, he stared across the room, at an eye chart on the wall, and began reading.

"A, E, X, D, R …"

The board was confused.

"The operation Dr. Kelman performed two days ago was on a certain Abe Levin." The man now smiled broadly. "I am Abe Levin, and I can see perfectly well with that eye."

The physicians on the board stared at Levin in disbelief, then stared at Kelman. They proceeded to examine his eyes and recheck his sight.

Levin's right macula had been healthier than his left. When Kelman had gone to examine him the day after surgery, Levin had been reading the newspaper in his bed.

This was irrefutable proof. The board found in Kelman's favor. Abe Levin had gained his sight, plus a brand new suit that Kelman had bought him from Bloomingdale's.

Kelman's success was unquestionable. He could extract a cataract through an incision that was one tenth the size of the conventional way. But, as he expected, many establishment doctors opposed him. By 1973, older ophthalmologists were beginning to lose cases to

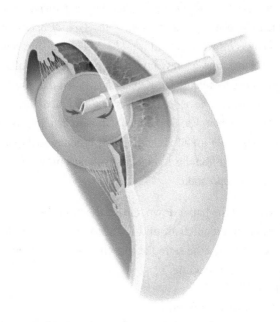

Phacoemulsification.

younger surgeons who had learned phacoemulsification. Some of the former criticized Kelman and his innovative procedure publicly, stating: "Phaco is OK after you learn it, but the first 50 eyes are blinded during the learning curve," or "Phaco causes glaucoma."

Kelman did not shrink from his detractors. To some, he quipped, "Anyone over age 30 is too old to learn phaco." He reveled in discharging his patients on the same day as surgery and letting them resume activities the next day, while most of his peers were keeping their patients hospitalized for a week. Often, the eyes looked so good after surgery that it didn't even look like any surgery had been performed.

Kelman published his work, and as he'd dreamed of doing, presented at the Academy meeting. Now *he* was on the podium. Other surgeons sought his counsel and he taught courses so they could learn the technique. Cavitron manufactured the phacoemulsification machine, which sold very well. It was called the "Kelman machine," and Charley Kelman became a very wealthy man.

In later years, he was able to devote more time to his music – singing and playing saxophone on stage. He gave a benefit concert at Carnegie Hall, and appeared on *The Tonight Show* with Johnny Carson. He gained notoriety by operating on famous people and commuting to Manhattan by helicopter, piloting himself. In 1992, he received the National Medal of Technology from President George H. W. Bush. His technique was later used by neurosurgeons to carefully extract tumors from the brain and spinal cord in children. Because he was the first in medicine to remove tissue through a small incision, some have credited him with inspiring the revolution in small-incision, laparoscopic surgery that came after him.

In 1962, a leader in the field had famously said, "Cataract surgery has been developed to its ultimate state, and any improvements from this date will be insignificant." Fortunately, Kelman thought otherwise, and almost everyone who's had cataract surgery in the last twenty-five years has benefited from his phacoemulsification technique.

Charles Kelman died on June 1, 2004. Phacoemulsification has now been performed on millions of people around the globe. It is the most commonly performed surgery in the world; perhaps it will one day become the most commonly performed surgery in human history. Through hard work, ingenuity, and persistence, Kelman achieved success, respect, and the quixotic thing he had wanted since he was a little boy – fame.

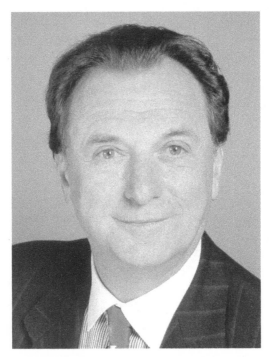

Charles Kelman, M.D.
Courtesy of the Albert and Mary Lasker Foundation.

Chapter Four | *"I did not want to be considered a military hero."*

CHARLES SCHEPENS AND THE BINOCULAR INDIRECT OPHTHALMOSCOPE

P hiladelphia 2006, *a Friday night*

"Hello?" I answer my cell phone and glance at the clock. *1 a.m.*

"Hi, Andrew? This is Evelyn in the ER."

"Yes, what is it?"

"I'm taking a referral…from a doctor on a cruise ship."

"What?"

"Yeah, it's in the Caribbean and I wasn't sure if I should accept the patient. There's a guy on the ship, he's from here, but they're on vacation and he's seeing flashes in his right eye."

"So they're calling us? Now?" I don't have the energy to make this a teachable moment for Evelyn. Sure, at worst, seeing flashes might mean that the vitreous gel in the center of the eye is pulling away from and tugging the retina; the tugging causes a flash, and if it pulls hard enough, it can result in a retinal tear. But lots of people get flashes, and the odds of a retinal tear are still low. It hardly warrants a middle-of-the-night consultation. "He needs to see an eye doctor. Try to find one the next place they stop," I say sleepily.

"He doesn't want to do that. He's had a retinal detachment in his other eye already – that didn't go well, his vision's legally blind in that eye. The symptoms here are the same as he had in the other eye. He's really nervous."

"So he wants to come here? Sure, alright. Accept it. If he gets here, I'll see him tomorrow."

"Ok, thanks. He's already called for a helicopter to take him from St. Thomas to San Juan first thing in the morning. Then he can fly here. Sorry to wake you."

I go back to bed.

Saturday night

"Hello?" I answer my cell phone and look at the clock. *1 a.m.*

"Hi Andrew? This is Tony in the ER."

"Tony? What is it?"

"There's a patient here who says he's supposed to see you. He, uh, came right from the airport. From a cruise ship in the Caribbean."

"He came *now*? I thought he was going to come during the day."

"Yeah, well, he's here. Looks like he's been through a lot."

I can hear myself sigh. "OK, why don't you take a look and call me if it's really something."

"Hello?" I answer my cell phone and look at the clock. *2 a.m.*

"Hi Andrew? Tony again."

"Yeah."

"This guy has a retinal tear."

"Any retinal detachment?"

"No, but there might be a little subretinal fluid around it."

I groan. "Alright, I'm coming in."

We are a world famous institution, but the Eye Emergency Room looks like it hasn't been updated in thirty years – because it hasn't. The walls are tan and vapid. The linoleum floor is dark and stained from decades of scuffs and spills. The teal cabinets and pink chart bins remind me of pictures I've seen of the hospital JFK died in.

The patient is waiting for me. He's wearing a suit and looks like he could be an executive. He's sweating and clearly distressed.

"Hi, I'm Doctor Lam." I shake his hand. "Sounds like you've had a very long day."

The suit man nods. "Thank you so much for seeing me, Doctor. I know this is an inconvenient time."

I nod. *Can't be mad at him now.*

"Let's take a look."

I pull a headset over my head and tighten it. The headset is a binocular indirect ophthalmoscope, used to see inside the eye and examine the peripheral retina. It's called an *indirect* ophthalmoscope because the image you obtain from it is a virtual image, suspended in mid-air and oriented upside-down, as opposed to a *direct* image, which would be a true image of the physical thing you're looking at and arranged right-side up. I adjust my eye pieces, which are actually prisms that take the lines of sight from each of my eyes and bring them so close together that they can both fit through the small space that is the pupil of the patient's eye, giving me a vivid, three-dimensional view inside. I hold a thick, round, twenty-diopter lens between me and his eye, using it to focus the image.

His retina has an orange glow. The optic nerve, which connects the eye to the brain, appears yellow and normal. The arteries and veins that emanate from the center of the optic nerve spread out and reach like tendrils to the outer periphery. This patient has some blood floating in his right eye; the wisps of red mix with the viscous vitreous gel like egg whites in a bowl of egg drop soup.

I see the tear at 12 o'clock, a big one.

He's 20/20 in the eye I'm examining, and 20/200 in the other eye, which shows lots of scarring from previous retina surgery. I take off the indirect ophthalmoscope and sit down.

"Well sir, you've got a retinal tear."

I start the talk I must give half-a-dozen times each week, mindful that for each patient, the subject is usually a new and frightening one.

"The retina is like the wallpaper lining the inside of your eye. You need it to be flat against the eye wall to see. There's a gel in the eye called the vitreous and it's normal in life for this gel to pull away from the retina. When this happens sometimes collagen fibers within the gel become opaque and cast shadows on the retina, which you may perceive as a floater. If the vitreous pulls hard enough on the retina, it can cause a *retinal tear,* which is bad because fluid in the eye can then go through the tear and get under the retina, 'ripping the wallpaper off the wall,' so to speak. That would be called a *retinal detachment.* When you get a detachment, you start to lose vision."

He's heard it all before but he's concentrating hard on every word I say.

"Right now you have a retinal tear but not a detachment. I can do a laser treatment which will help the retina stick to the eye wall. It will significantly reduce the risk of a detachment."

He nods. We talk a little more, I answer his questions, and he signs the consent form.

I perform the laser treatment using another indirect ophthalmoscope with a laser attachment mounted on the front of it.

Inside the eye I see a tiny red dot, the *aiming beam,* in the middle of my circle of light, and when I step on the pedal and hold it down, the laser fires repeatedly, emitting bright green pulses. Each laser spot makes a retinal burn which will become a scar that adheres the retina to the eye wall. I surround the retinal tear with laser burns. It only takes a couple minutes. Unlike in phacoemulsification surgery, a history of playing video games helps a lot with the hand-eye coordination required for this procedure.

I follow the patient's progress over the next few months. The laser scars look good. He does not develop a retinal detachment, his vision is saved, and he continues his work without interruption.

One man's invention allowed my operation to be a successful, even routine, one. His name was Charles Schepens, and he invented the binocular indirect ophthalmoscope – an instrument that revolutionized our ability to diagnose and treat diseases located inside the eye.

The first time I saw the retina through the indirect ophthalmoscope, I gasped. It was incredibly beautiful. There had only been a few similar awe-inspiring moments in my life, times when I thought to myself, "God did not intend for us to be here, seeing this." It happened the first time I saw a beating heart and held it in my hands during cardiac surgery. The same feeling when the patient came off the bypass machine and I shocked the heart back to life with paddles. It's surreal, but it's real.

For me, seeing the retina in vivid, three-dimensional detail was like that. It takes a while for a medical student to learn to see the retina well; in fact, many non-ophthalmologists can't do it. At first, we're trained to use something called a direct ophthalmoscope in medical school. You've seen it, the flashlight stick with a keyhole fitting on top which your primary care doctor holds very close to your face. They're very difficult to use well unless the eye is dilated, something rarely done outside an eye doctor's office. The exercise sometimes just shows you if your doctor has *halitosis* – bad breath.

What really allows you to see the retina well is either a slit-lamp, the microscope mounted on a small table at the eye doctor's office, or an indirect ophthalmoscope. In both methods, focusing lenses are used to bring the back of the eye into focus.

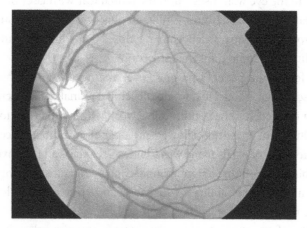

A view of normal retina showing the optic nerve and macula.

© 2002 American Academy of Ophthalmology.

The retina is light-sensing tissue that lines the inside of the eye like the film in a camera; it's really part of the neurological system, a distant component of the brain. When there is systemic disease, you can see all sorts of things going haywire in the retina. In diabetics, blood vessels burst, leak, and bleed. If a clot stops blood flow to the retina, you can see the tissue whiten and die right before your eyes. There's even a parasite, a worm, that likes to migrate to the retina; it can sometimes be seen crawling around, leaving tracks all over the place. The luckiest trainees get a chance to zap the worm with a laser, killing it.

The retinal problem most people have heard of is a retinal

detachment. This condition undoubtedly caused many cases of unexplained blindness prior to the mid-twentieth century – unexplained because of an inability to diagnose problems residing inside the eye. The *direct* ophthalmoscope was invented in 1853, by a German ophthalmologist named Herman Helmholtz, but it wasn't until Charles Schepens invented the *binocular indirect ophthalmoscope* that we really began to see the retina well. This instrument finally enabled doctors to diagnose retinal detachments and begin to devise treatments to fix them. This is why Schepens is called the "Father of modern retinal surgery."

Among ophthalmologists, Dr. Schepens is world-famous for his contributions to the field. He built his career in Boston, where the Institute he founded bears his name. But what many ophthalmologists find most fascinating about this giant of our field is not his medical accomplishments, but something totally non-medical – something he did as a young man during World War II. Dr. Schepens was usually reticent about his former life because he feared the story would overshadow his medical accomplishments; but it is a story that must be told, for it illustrates the qualities of a man who would make the world a better place.

JULY 21, 1943 *Mendive, France*

The toes of Jacques Perot's leather boots were leaking again. He could feel the tips of his socks growing more damp with each padded step on the moss-carpeted forest floor. The wetness annoyed him, and this feeling brought back memories of his other life, his previous life, and his resentment for the Germans swelled anew.

He took a deep breath.

Ankle-high mist clung to the floor of the Foret d'Iraty, in the Pyrenees. Small white mushroom caps dotted the almost indiscernible trail. Overhead, the orange glow of dawn was beginning to suffuse the tall fir trees, century-old spruces, and hemlocks.

Perot tried to still the confusion of moods and thoughts in his mind. In his heart he was an optimist, and he let the good memories of the past flash before his mind – the comfortable townhome in Brussels, his wife Cette running after their two children in the park, his predictable daily work as an ophthalmologist, and his leisure time devoted to pondering the eye's mysteries and the ways to improve seeing inside it. All this seemed so long ago to him now.

A stoat darted across his path, disappearing into a hole underneath a rotten log. He chuckled to himself. A year ago the sudden animal would have startled him – being a city dweller. But now when he hiked through the woods he almost imagined himself a woodsman. After all, he was the manager of a lumber mill. If his old friends and colleagues could see him now…he was sure they were where he had left them, attending to their lives in German-occupied Belgium. The war probably hadn't changed *them* very much.

Had they any idea what had become of Charles Schepens? That was Perot's real name. And, if one of his friends were to see him… what then? Was he recognizable?

No one knew he'd joined the Belgian underground. Nor that, for the past year, he'd been managing a sawmill on the border between France and Spain, a sawmill that was a front to get refugees out of occupied France.

Perot fully believed in what he was doing, but even so, it was hard on Cette and the children, Luc and Claire. That part he didn't like.

As part of his cover, he did his best to ingratiate himself with the local Gestapo, expressing friendship, encouraging them to visit him, plying them with gifts of wine, cheese, and other carefully rationed foodstuffs. He played this role so well that the local townsfolk and even most of his employees thought he was a collaborator. The locals could not risk offending him since he was the man who employed dozens of workers. Yet it pained him that they treated Cette and the children badly because of his friendliness with the Germans. This, Perot accepted, was part of the job of helping others to survive.

Cette, herself, did not guess the true purpose of the mill, and it never really came up in any of their conversations. However, every month a dozen "temporary" workers disappeared from the mill and were led over the border by shepherds loyal to the cause. These were workers who were actually downed Allied pilots, resistance fighters with bounties on their heads, or Jews. If Cette sensed any of this was the case, she never let on.

The sun was fully up now, the forest filled with light. Perot quickened his steps toward home. It was important to make sure the mill was up and running, the loggers were done with breakfast and on their way to work, and the quirky cable system that pulled the logs out of the valley was operating properly.

Nearing the town, Perot heard sudden footfalls on the slick trail. It was Nicolas, his assistant. It was not like Nicolas to take to the woods. He was an accountant and his body was made for a chair. But now, with one look at the man, Perot knew something had happened.

"Jacques!" Nicolas said all out of breath.

"What's wrong?" Perot questioned in French. "Is it Cette?"

The little man shook his head. "It's...the...Gestapo!"

Nicolas pointed down to the clearing below, part of the town of Lecumberry, where he and many of the workers lived.

Perot took a deep breath.

"At my house?"

"No, at the factory."

The factory was in Mendive, the adjacent town, a short distance away. He had a little time.

"What do they want?"

"They won't say. They will only talk to you. I said you were not available, but..."

"Yes?"

"They said they'd wait."

"How long has it been?"

"At least an hour. And they're from Paris."

Damn, Perot thought. *They came this early?* He was used to the local Gestapo, normally somewhat amiable, often a little lazy and quite comfort-seeking. Perot knew they felt lucky to be stationed in this little corner of France, away from the action, and he'd never known them to be early risers. No, these Gestapo were a different breed. From Paris. This was serious.

First he thought of Cette and the children. *Better not alarm them. See what the Germans want, then make decisions, if necessary.*

"Don't worry, Nicolas. See to your duties, I'll go meet them."

Nicolas nodded.

Perot walked to the end of the trail and turned right on the narrow hard-packed dirt road, toward Mendive. He wondered what Nicolas knew of their secret operation. Very few knew the true purpose of the mill. He, himself, insisted on never meeting the refugees. It was safer that way. None of the saved actually knew who he was.

A shiny black sedan with yellow wheels was parked in front of the office, a one-room, wood-planked building. He could see four tall men standing around the car, smoking cigarettes. They were wearing plain clothes, which was typical for Gestapo.

They turned to face him as he approached.

Perot forced a smile.

"Good morning, Gentlemen," he said in German with a small bow.

One of them, a stout man with an arrogant air, came up to him. Like the rest of them, he wore a collared shirt and tie, and pleated trousers – apparel more suited to a banker than a man of action. Perot was wearing his usual workday khaki shirt and shorts.

"Good morning, Monsieur Perot," the front man said, studying him closely. The other three casually but deliberately surrounded him while also eyeing the workers who stopped to stare on their way to the saw mill. For a moment Perot's eyes fell to the Gestapos' shiny black boots, the only part of their dress that was military. He looked at his own canvas espadrilles, and realized how unprepared he was for a fight, or a run.

"How can I help you gentlemen?"

"Your German is quite good," the leader said.

Perot smiled.

"I will come straight to the point. A man has been arrested who says you've been passing people into Spain. He says this has been happening for some time now, and that you receive money from outside France to keep this little operation of yours going."

"That's ridiculous, who is the man who tells these lies?"

The Gestapo officer waved his hand dismissively. "That isn't your concern. What else would you like to say for yourself?"

Perot's heart pounded. It must have been Vallier, the new courier sent from London with funds from the exiled Belgian government. Perot had worried about him from the moment they'd met a few weeks before – the man joked too much; he was the type who thought this was all just an adventure, a game.

"You should ask around. Any local German official will tell you that nothing could be farther from the truth. In fact, I have orders I can show you that prove the lumber from our mill is used for the defense of France from an Allied invasion!"

Perot eyed the men. Their disposition was unknown. But there was a darkness around them.

The four Gestapo agents were silent for several seconds. The smell of fresh cut resinous lumber wafted over from the mill, and the sound of the saw whining, the rotation belt slapping, came and went as the big logs passed through. Then the agent in charge turned and spoke to his men in a low voice.

Perot could not hear him. He tried to assume an impatient, yet dignified stance. It was important to look a bit indignant, he thought, but not disrespectful. Everything hinged on what they said next.

The Gestapo leader turned on his heel. "It's obvious," he said, "you're put out by this unexpected visit. Don't be nervous. We've decided to believe you."

Perot felt a head rush of relief.

The German opened a cigarette case, snapped a small gold lighter, and drew the smoke into his lungs. Exhaling through his nose, he spoke softly, so that Perot had to lean forward to hear him. "Yes, but most unfortunately, we shall have to bring you to Paris to answer some questions…in a more formal setting. We do apologize for the inconvenience."

Perot bit his tongue. There was no way he was getting into that car.

"I see," he said. "Well, if you insist." Then he gazed around, as if worried about the mill. "But please, gentlemen, you must allow me a little time. We have over a hundred workers here and I must see that things go smoothly in my absence. We don't want to hold up the lumber needed for the Wehrmacht's defense…do we?" He let this thought settle in.

The German officer glanced at his wristwatch. "Very well. But I must warn you to be quick about it."

Perot nodded and, though he wanted to sprint, walked to the opposite side of the mill, where he would be hidden from their view. He found Nicolas hiding in a corner.

"Nicolas. Cut the telephone lines out of here. They know who I am. I've got to escape to Spain. Tell Cette to meet me with the children at the border."

He didn't have time to explain further, but he hoped that Nicolas would do exactly as he asked. He turned from the younger man and darted into the woods. He would head for the border. He didn't look back.

That misty morning in July 1943 was a defining moment in Charles Schepens' life. He had truly dedicated himself to his secret life at the saw mill. In later years, he wrote, "At the time, I even had the idea that I could spend the balance of my life there, give up medicine, and get a diploma from some forestry department." If Schepens' story had ended here, he would be remembered as a brave hero of the Resistance; but remarkably, it was for what he later accomplished in the field of ophthalmology that humanity owes him the greatest debt.

Schepens was a Belgian ophthalmologist in Brussels when the Germans invaded his country in May 1940. He was apolitical by nature, but in October 1940, Gestapo agents came to his office and accused him of helping Allied pilots escape the country. They ransacked his office and threw him in prison for ten days. The charges were false, but the episode spurred him to action against the Germans.

He subsequently allowed his office to serve as a drop site for the Resistance, where secret documents and money could be deposited before being smuggled out of the country. Schepens' biographer, Meg Ostrum, writes, "Every few weeks a Flemish-speaking 'patient' would make an appointment and bring along a brown satchel filled with secret documents that he hid in the thick ivy on the wall at the rear of the property," until the Resistance could pick it up.

He continued these activities until April 1942, when he got advance word that he was under surveillance. He immediately fled to France and assumed a new name, Jacques Perot. He continued to work for the Belgian Resistance network, and agreed to rebuild and manage the sawmill in the Pyrenees on the border between France and Spain. He helped more than a hundred Resistance fighters, Jews and Allied airmen escape capture by the Nazis. He also facilitated the passing of secret documents in and out of occupied France.

After his last-minute escape that fateful morning in 1943, Schepens trekked in the Pyrenees for several days, ultimately crossing the border and arriving at San Sebastian. He learned his wife and children were being kept under house arrest; the Gestapo hoped he would attempt a rescue, so they could trap him. Though it pained him not to try, Schepens knew such an attempt would be foolhardy. In October 1943, the Belgian underground based in London provided the funds and necessary paperwork for him to go to England. Later that same month, the Germans began to relax their surveillance of his family, and with the help of other Belgian agents, Cette, Claire and Luc, who were aged five and three, respectively, made good their own escape from France. Their long journey included hiking through the Pyrenees, transport by bicycle, days spent hiding in the back of a truck, and nights spent outdoors in thunderstorms. After nine months of separation, Cette and the children made it to London and were re-united with Schepens.

Near the end of the war Schepens worked at Moorfields Eye Hospital in London, where he'd previously trained as a registrar (resident). This was the same illustrious eye hospital where Harold Ridley had worked. Later, Schepens recalled, "When I looked inside the patients' eyes at Moorfields, I was very frustrated when I thought I detected a detached retina, but I couldn't really see it in three-dimensional relief with the monoscope. The idea of an ophthalmoscope that would enable doctors to look with both eyes at the retina possessed me, although none of my superiors at Moorfields believed it was possible to construct such a device."

The main problem with getting the stereoscopic view he wanted was a human dilemma – we need both eyes to see in three-dimensions, but our eyes are spaced too far apart to use together when trying to see through a space with the diameter of another person's pupil. Furthermore, even if one could solve the problem of using both eyes to see through such a tiny space, there is the additional challenge of having a light source strong enough to be transmitted along the line of sight to illuminate the retina inside.

Schepens experimented with prisms and mirrors, trying to find a way to take the examiner's lines of sight from each eye and bring them closer together, close enough so that both could squeeze through the pupil. To do this, he devised an apparatus that positioned a prism in front of each eye. Each prism bent the line of sight from each eye toward the nose. In the middle, right in front of the nose, there were two more prisms next to one another. These prisms bent the sight lines out, straight ahead, so that the sight lines from each eye were adjacent to each other, almost touching. He mounted the apparatus on a headband and positioned himself directly underneath a powerful light. A mirror reflected the light straight out, along the same axis as his line of sight.

With this unwieldy apparatus on his head, Schepens held a magnifying lens between him and the eye of his subject. Suddenly, he saw an aerial view of the retina. It was upside down. Right and left were reversed. But the image was large, vivid, and three-dimensional! He had created a virtual, "indirect" image.

Schepens built this rudimentary prototype in 1945, using pieces of scrap metal he'd found after scouring the site of a building that had been hit by a V-2 rocket. In later models he attached the light source to the headband itself.

After the war, Schepens returned to Belgium and reestablished his practice of ophthalmology. He was dedicated to developing new and improved tools to better examine the retina, but he soon became frustrated by the lack of scientific inquiry in his own country. It became clear that he would have to leave Europe if he was to achieve his scientific goals, and that the place to go was America, the country most conducive to research. In 1947, Schepens went to Boston and perfected his ophthalmoscope. He founded the Retina Foundation in 1950, which was later re-named the Schepens Eye Research Institute. Today it is the largest independent eye research institute in the world. Schepens' subsequent research on surgery for retinal detachments increased the success rate of reattachment from 40% to 90%.

During his lifetime, Schepens preferred not to be recognized for his wartime activities. He did not want attention from this to draw away from his achievements in ophthalmology, which he considered his true legacy and contribution to mankind. "I did not want to be considered a military hero," he said.

Charles Schepens died in 2006, at the age of ninety-four.

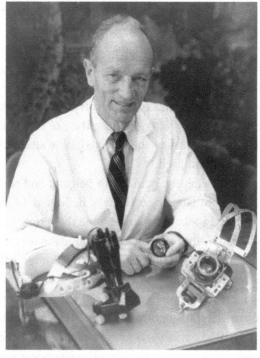

Charles Schepens, M.D., with an indirect ophthalmoscope (left) and an early prototype (right).

Courtesy of the Schepens Eye Research Institute.

I use Schepens' indirect ophthalmoscope fifty times a day in my practice. Without it, I would be of little use to my patients. With it, I see their retinas in vivid, living color and can identify problems invisible to practitioners before the mid-twentieth century.

For millennia, there was no way to diagnose or treat a retinal detachment. One could see the retina with the direct ophthalmoscope, which was invented in the mid-nineteenth century, but with it, it was difficult to have confidence in diagnosing a detachment and practically impossible to accurately locate the retinal tear or tears that caused it. Primitive early treatments for detachments included compressive bandages, bed rest, pilocarpine injections, mercury ointment, electrolysis, and retinal sutures. All of these were almost completely ineffective.

A Swiss ophthalmologist named Jules Gonin was the first to understand that retinal detachments were precipitated by a hole or tear in the retina. In 1920, he began to treat detachments by cauterizing the sclera, the white outer coat of the eye, over where the tear was localized. Of course, at the time this was very difficult because of poor visualization with the direct ophthalmoscope. Imagine you are looking through the pupil as you would through a keyhole. You have a small flashlight and are peering into a large room. You move your head this way and that, trying to search the ceiling, the floor, while you are pressed up against the door, in reality less than an inch from the patient's face. You think you see something way up in a dark corner of the room, perhaps a tear in the wallpaper. Then you step back and get your cautery probe. You then *estimate* where you think the tear may be, and cauterize the sclera. You can imagine that this is usually less than accurate. The tear might be less than a millimeter in size. And what's worse, Gonin's treatments actually involved *intentionally* perforating the sclera, allowing the fluid under the retina to leak out, and then attempting to contact the actual underside of the retinal hole or tear, to cauterize it. Amazingly, he reported a 53% success rate. Later surgeons realized that cauterizing just the scleral surface over the tear could be effective.

The next surgical advance was the scleral buckle, first performed in 1937. The fact that we still do this type of surgery today is a testament to its effectiveness. Dr. Schepens did much to improve this procedure. The "buckle" is a silicone band that is sutured tightly to the sclera, indenting the eye wall. Think of this as a way to bring the wall of a room closer in, making it easier to reattach the wallpaper. Techniques improved with the use of cryotherapy, the freezing treatment Charles Kelman investigated, in place of "hot" thermal cautery. Later advancements included the injection of gas bubbles in the eye, which float upward and, depending on how the patient positions his or her head, can push the retina back against the eye wall.

Finally, the type of surgery that I do most often was developed. It is called a *vitrectomy*, because it involves removal of the vitreous gel. Like the appendix, this gel serves no useful purpose, except to cause problems like retinal tears. The vitrector instrument was developed by Dr. Robert Machemer in 1971, and is a small, thin probe that is inserted into the eye, where it sucks vitreous gel into a port, while a cutter inside the port chops the gel at a rate of up to 2500 cuts per minute. This rapid cutting is very important because if one were to simply suck or pull on the vitreous, this would exert traction on the retina and might cause several retinal tears right away. Amazingly, Machemer built his first vitrector using a simple plastic syringe and a AA battery.

Now I can perform a vitrectomy to repair a retinal detachment in about thirty minutes. Our instruments are inserted through tiny holes made through the sclera near the front of the eye. These small incisions heal on their own – no sutures are needed. In the surgery we clear out the vitreous, flatten the retina by filling the eye with air, use a fiberoptic laser probe to laser-seal the area of the tear precisely, and finally fill the eye with a gas bubble that lasts for several weeks. The gas bubble keeps the retina pressed against the eye wall long enough for the detachment to heal, and gradually gets absorbed into the bloodstream on its own. What was before a blinding disease is now usually successfully repaired with restoration of vision.

To a retinal surgeon like me, Charles Schepens is the Thomas Edison, Charles Lindbergh, and Henry Ford of our field. It would be impossible to effectively fix retinal detachments without his invention. The original prototype of his ophthalmoscope is on display at the Smithsonian Institution. He was a courageous and inventive man. If he hadn't first escaped Belgium, and then occupied France, he would not have invented his indirect ophthalmoscope and tens of thousands might still be going blind from retinal detachments today.

Chapter Five | *"…eighteen out of twenty-one…"*

ARNALL PATZ, RETINOPATHY OF PREMATURITY, AND A LOOMING CRISIS

I picked up the ringing phone in my office.

"Hi Andrew. Sorry to bother you. I was wondering if you could take a look at a baby in the NICU." It was the pediatric ophthalmologist calling from the neonatal intensive care unit. This doctor screened premature babies for *retinopathy of prematurity* or *ROP.*

"Sure, tell me about it."

I heard him sigh. "This one's progressed quickly. He was born at twenty-three weeks – "

I whistled.

" – I know, believe me, I know. I'm amazed he's made it this far. He's at thirty-six weeks now. Poor kid's already been to Boston for PDA surgery and another surgery here for nec."

I recalled the terms from medical school: *patent ductus arteriosis* – failure of an embryonic blood vessel to close normally after birth, resulting in abnormal blood flow between the aorta and pulmonary artery; *necrotizing enterocolitis* – death of the inner lining of the digestive tract, related to inadequate blood flow or possibly bacteria.

It was my turn to sigh. A full term baby is born 40 weeks after the mother's last menstrual period. This baby, born at the cusp of viability, still had yet to reach the 40 week mark.

I kept listening.

"Like I said, it's going quick. It didn't look too bad when I saw him just about a week ago, but now it's definite stage 3 with plus disease."

"Retina flat?"

"I think so. I don't see a detachment, but there's some hemorrhage that makes it hard to see. I'd feel better if you took a look at it. He might need a laser treatment."

"Sure, what's the name and bed number? I'll come over and check him out."

A NICU is like no other place in the hospital. You gain entry through heavy, locked doors after showing the front desk clerk your ID. You are confronted by a bank of huge sinks, like the ones outside an operating room, and signs command you to scrub your hands for at least two minutes. After drying your hands, you enter a surreal world of low hanging fluorescent lights, hushed voices, and rows and rows of tiny plastic boxes called isolettes, which house premature babies. Some of the babies are wearing eye masks under glowing blue lights, like clients of a tanning salon, except that they're getting specialized light treatment to break down the toxic bilirubin that is still floating in their bloodstreams.

If you venture close to one of the isolettes, you'll find a tiny miracle inside. Actually, as any parent would tell you, each baby is a *huge* miracle – in a tiny body. Our ever-improving ability to keep these premature newborns alive outside the womb is a triumph of modern medicine. In your hands, the babies seem impossibly small, and when you see the IVs and other miniature tubes coming out of them, it's easy to feel overwhelmed by the multitude of medical problems each one faces in their fight for survival. Yet beside each one, there is usually a mother or young couple, holding a vigil, desperately praying their baby will grow, mature, and live. For all these reasons, the NICU can be both the most depressing and uplifting place in a hospital.

The baby I went to see that afternoon was named Danny. The nurse had to tell me this, because Danny's bracelet only said, "Baby Boy," next to the parents' last name. I introduced myself to Danny's parents. Dad was a writer. Mom was a teacher – a kindergarten teacher. I explained why I needed to look into Danny's eyes, to check for retinopathy of prematurity, and asked them to wait for me in the family waiting area.

Danny was sleeping peacefully, encased in his plastic box with two round doors in the side which could be opened to permit grown-ups to place their hands inside. The progress notes said he weighed four pounds, which was impressive, given he'd only weighed one and a half pounds at birth. He was just over a foot long; his tiny arms had the diameter of my thumb.

The nurse helped me to slide Danny out of the isolette. I put a numbing eye drop in each eye. He'd been given drops to dilate his pupils an hour before, but as I slid a small metal speculum between the eyelids of his right eye, to hold them open, I noticed his pupils were still fairly small.

"Did you put the drops in an hour ago?"

The nurse nodded.

I used a flashlight to get a better look. Danny was awake now, and not happy; he squirmed and cried as the nurse kept him tightly swaddled and held his head still for me. There was a thin web of blood vessels all around the rim of the pupil – *neovascularization,* an abnormal sign indicative of severe ROP and the reason the normally flexible iris tissue was not dilating well.

It was going to be a tough view inside the eye.

I put on my indirect ophthalmoscope and peered through the pupil to examine Danny's retina.

Blood, I saw immediately. I remembered what the pediatric ophthalmologist had said. *He wasn't kidding.*

A thin red mist of hemorrhage clouded the view generally, and there were patches of dense blood globs that looked like dripped red paint overlying parts of the retinal periphery. I could see, at least, that the retina was flat and not detached. There was a well-demarcated border between the vascularized retina which had developed normally, and the more peripheral, white retina where the growing blood vessels had yet to reach. Many fronds of neovascularization rose up along the border between these two zones of vascular and avascular retina, and there was obvious *plus disease,* a term used to describe the dilated and tortuous blood vessels in the back of the eye that indicate advanced ROP.

The other eye looked about the same.

"Definite laser," I muttered under my breath as I gently removed the speculum from Danny's eyelids.

"What?" the nurse asked, not hearing me.

I cleared my throat and said more clearly, "He's got severe ROP and needs a laser treatment. The peripheral retina isn't vascularized and those areas are sending out signals for the retina to grow new vessels."

"What's wrong with that?"

I smiled. This nurse asked good questions.

"The new vessels that grow are abnormal. They bleed and form fibrotic membranes that can pull on the retina and cause a

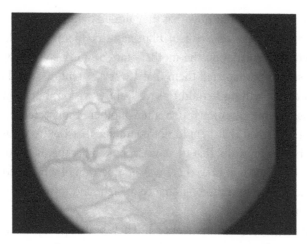

A view of peripheral retina in Stage 3 Retinopathy of Prematurity. Normal blood vessel development has been arrested; neovascularization is present at the border between vascular (left side) and avascular (right side) retina.

© 2002 American Academy of Ophthalmology.

retinal detachment. If I laser the peripheral, non-vascular areas, the signaling will stop, and so will the abnormal neovascularization."

"But won't the laser hurt his vision?"

"Well, the areas I need to laser aren't developed – they're already non-functioning. If we don't do it, the abnormal vessels are likely to keep growing and there's a good chance his retinas will detach. Then he might end up completely blind."

What I didn't tell the nurse was that blood was obscuring my view of several areas I needed to laser. At best, this would be partial treatment.

I hoped it would be enough.

I spent a long time talking to Danny's parents. They'd already been through two surgeries for life-threatening problems. Until this point, they hadn't even considered that their son's eyes could also be a problem, but now that they understood the gravity of the situation, the very real risk of blindness hit them hard. Halfway through my explanation the mother started to cry softly. I wanted to pause and perhaps tell them that I was a parent, too, and that I would do everything I could to save Danny's vision, but the father kept asking me questions, one after another. I answered each of them. I explained that I could not guarantee that Danny would see well when he grew up, that there was a possibility that he would see poorly, but that right now, there was no question of what needed to be done to give him the best chance at sight and to prevent retinal detachment in both eyes.

Finally, the questions stopped. They both had tears running down their cheeks.

I promised to do my best.

Retinopathy of prematurity was not a problem that got much attention before the mid-twentieth century. This was simply because up until the 1940s, very premature babies usually didn't survive. When we are small embryos, the blood vessels that will nourish our retinas begin to grow out of the center of the optic nerve at the back of the eye. As the weeks in the womb go by, the vessels grow further and further out into the retinal periphery – it takes almost the entire forty weeks of a normal pregnancy for the retina to become fully vascularized. When a baby is born prematurely, the process is cut short, and for a baby born as early as twenty-three weeks gestation, those tiny, sight-giving vessels still have a really long way to go.

Most of the time, the blood vessels still *do* develop and the baby's retina can be normal. All along, the undeveloped, unvascularized segments of the retina are sending out a molecule called *vascular endothelial growth factor,* or *VEGF,* for short, which is a special signal that promotes vessel growth. The problem is, this proliferation of VEGF above normal levels causes abnormally prolific vessel growth. Like unwanted weeds in a garden, the resulting *neovascular* vessels form wispy, fragile webs that rise from the retina and invest themselves into the vitreous gel that fills the eye. These vessels are immature and apt to bleed, and the webs can coalesce to form fibrous membranes that contract and pull on the retina, causing a detachment.

If you're amazed that anyone could have figured out this complex disease process, which happens inside the tiny eyes of the smallest human bodies, I'd tell you I feel the same way. It wasn't until after World War II that Charles Schepens' invention of the indirect ophthalmoscope allowed retina specialists to view the retina in full, so it's no surprise that ophthalmologists of the mid-twentieth century had no clue that a blinding disease process was occurring inside these babies' eyes. In fact, there was no outward sign of a problem at all until a total retinal detachment occurred, at which time the retina was lifted so far forward that it was easily seen as a sheet of dead, white tissue behind the pupil. This explains why this curiosity was first given a generic, descriptive name: *retrolental fibroplasia.*

It's also easy to understand why most NICU doctors in the immediate post-war period might not have given much thought to the eye. Confronted with a room full of premature babies, each with a slew of life-threatening problems, it's natural that they wouldn't consider the eye a top priority.

But thank God one man did.

———

Arnall Patz, as his friends described him, was a kind and modest man. Throughout his long career, he seemed incapable of guile or politicking. But beneath this serene exterior was a man with great ambition – though not for himself. His ambition was to save the sight of others.

Patz was born in 1920, in rural Elberton, Georgia. He was the youngest of seven children, and perhaps his position in the family birth order explains something about his unselfish personality. Patz's father, a Jewish immigrant from Lithuania, had wandered into Elberton many years before, scraping out a living as a traveling peddler. He was surprised to find that the owner of the town's general store was also a Jew, and even more surprised when the man offered him a job. Mr. Patz happily gave up his nomadic way of life for the chance to put down roots.

As Arnall Patz grew up, he, too, put in many hours working at the general store. The Depression was on, and Patz knew he was one of the lucky ones. He had plenty to eat, attended school, and had a job at the store on the weekends. He found resourceful ways to explore his interest in science, by fashioning his own rudimentary camera out of a couple of loose lenses and an old cigar box, or closely examining onion skins with a magnifying glass. Small for his age, Patz made an easy target for bullies. Thankfully, his best friend, a much taller boy named Brown Thompson, stood up for him more than once. And it was Brown's father, Dr. Thompson, the town doctor, who first encouraged Patz to consider becoming a physician.

After attending Emory University for college and medical school, Patz joined the Army near the end of World War II. He was stationed at Camp Lee, Virginia. It has been said that, during this time, he was trying to decide whether to go into internal medicine or ophthalmology, and that it was his first assignment in the Army – inspecting returning servicemen for sexually transmitted diseases – that steered him away from medicine and toward ophthalmology. Sometimes, a very sick patient in the infirmary at Camp Lee required transfer to Walter Reed General Hospital in Washington, D.C. A doctor was required to monitor the patient during this four-hour ambulance ride and Patz volunteered to do this on several occasions.

During one visit to Walter Reed he learned of an assistant position in the eye clinic. The eye intrigued him, so he managed to get transferred to Washington so he could take the position. The next year, he started his ophthalmology residency at Gallinger Municipal Hospital, which later became the District of Columbia General Hospital.

One of his duties as a resident was to examine the premature babies in the NICU for retrolental fibroplasia, which would later be termed ROP. This disease was the leading cause of childhood blindness at the time; the same condition would later blind Stevie Wonder. When he arrived, Patz examined twenty-one babies with the disease, knowing there was little he could do for them. These tiny babies were already sentenced to a lifetime of blindness.

But then, Patz noticed something different about the babies. In those days, many doctors believed that most premature infants would benefit from continuous, high levels of oxygen. This oxygen was typically pumped through special tubing into the babies' airtight incubators. It was a logical idea: if an infants' lungs aren't fully developed, one would think extra oxygen would be helpful.

Except that Patz realized that eighteen of the twenty-one cases of retrolental fibroplasia had incubators fitted with the special tubing. One of the babies even had a folded cone of x-ray film secured to its face. *For what?* he wondered. Then he saw, it was to concentrate the oxygen even more. And that's when it hit him: eighteen out of twenty-one were getting extra-high levels of oxygen.

He wondered, could it be that the continuous oxygen was promoting this blinding disease?

When Patz examined the retinas of these babies, he saw the blood vessels were extremely narrow. They extended from the optic nerve and spread out into the retinal periphery like the roots of a tree stretching to cover more ground – but for some reason, the vessels had all at once stopped growing. The retina toward the back of the eye, which had already been vascularized, had an orange-red glow – it was *alive*. The retina beyond the reach of the blood vessels was stark white – avascular. *Dead.*

Patz watched these eyes closely. Once the blood vessels stopped growing, new webs of tiny, thin blood vessels began to grow up from the retina at the border between these vascular and avascular zones. Then, a few days later the blood vessels would bleed a little. Then they would bleed a lot. Perhaps a couple weeks later they might coalesce to form a fibrous membrane, which would contract, and then a retinal detachment would occur.

Patz didn't know why high levels of oxygen might cause this process, but he couldn't disregard what he'd observed. Eighteen out of twenty-one babies was a statistic he could not ignore.

Now, keep in mind that Patz was only a resident at this time, still in training and probably still working on perfecting his examination and diagnostic skills. But he was smart and thoughtful, and he knew the only way to find the answer to his question would be to conduct a clinical trial in which some babies got the elevated oxygen and other babies didn't – these babies could still have oxygen, of course, just not ultra-high, continuous amounts of it. At the same time, he knew that some doctors, perhaps all of them, would consider the idea of withholding high-level oxygen harmful, maybe even malpractice.

The first person Patz told his idea to was the pediatrician in charge of the nursery, Dr. Leroy Hoeck. To his relief, Hoeck agreed that Patz had made an important observation, and he wanted to help him organize a study trial to investigate it. The problem was, Hoeck didn't have any money to pay for the study.

But Patz was resourceful. Though he'd never written a grant proposal before, he decided to apply to the National Institutes of Health for a grant to conduct the trial. He asked for $4,000. He carefully wrote his proposal, sent it off, and waited.

His proposal was rejected. The NIH said his application was *unscientific*.

Most young residents would certainly have stopped there. Residents are not often encouraged to think outside the box or to challenge the status quo. Learning medicine, even more so then than now, was primarily an exercise in rote memorization in the lecture hall. Clinical experience was gained by observing senior doctors – if you observe a technique enough times, the theory went, you should be able to do it yourself. No one was showing Patz the ropes. He was making it up as he went along.

And he didn't stop.

He knew he had to do something to try to save the eyes of helpless babies like the ones he'd examined. If he didn't, no one else was going to. So he decided to borrow the $4,000 from his brother, who was running a successful trucking business, and he began the study.

Patz probably did not realize the significance of this simple act – of beginning his study – but his was the *first* randomized clinical trial in the field of ophthalmology to ever be done; in fact, it was among the first in all of medicine. Randomized clinical trials, in which patients are randomly assigned to one treatment or another, are the gold standard method of answering research questions. These studies are commonplace today, but in 1948, no ophthalmologist, much less a *resident,* had ever completed such a study.

As you might expect, there was open opposition to Patz's "experiment." Interestingly, the most dramatic example of this did not stem from his superiors, but from the NICU nurses. Some of them could not bring themselves to withhold what they thought was life-saving oxygen from the babies under their care; and, for a time, they secretly re-connected the tubing and gave high levels of oxygen to the babies who were not supposed to be getting it – at night, when no one was looking. Thankfully, this practice came to light and Patz spent more time explaining to the nurses what he had observed and why he was conducting the study. After this, the nurses got on board and all of them followed his protocol to the letter.

Patz studied the babies from 1948 to 1950. After the first year, his data showed that seven of the 28 babies who had received high levels of oxygen had developed ROP. None of the babies in the low oxygen group got the disease. He also demonstrated a clear and direct correlation between the number of days on high oxygen therapy and the incidence of ROP. In short, it looked like Patz might have made an amazing discovery.

At the same time, he tried to replicate the disease in an animal model, so he could conduct experiments and try to determine how oxygen toxicity might be causing the disease. He first tried using the opossum, partly because a veterinarian he knew recommended a trapper in South Carolina who could supply pregnant opossums. Patz exposed the resulting sixty-nine baby opossums to highly concentrated oxygen, but he soon regretted his choice of animal when he realized that opossum mothers were fiercely protective of their young. On recollecting these early days, he later wrote, "On one occasion while I was inserting an oxygen tube into the cage of the incubator to measure the oxygen concentration, the mother viciously snapped the tube approximately 1 mm distal to my index finger." Patz gave up on the opossum.

Next he turned to mice and dogs with greater success. As he exposed more and more animals to continuous, elevated oxygen and examined their retinas, he saw that high oxygen exposure first caused marked vasoconstriction of the peripheral retinal vessels, essentially closing them off and rendering them nonfunctional. Later on, the opposite would happen to the vessels that had previously developed in the back of the eye – these would become very dilated and tortuous, what was later classified as *plus disease*, and new tufts of capillary vessels began appearing at the border between the vascular and avascular zones of retina, the process later termed *neovascularization*. The clinical animal model looked just like what he'd seen in the premature babies with ROP.

Now he could be confident that the oxygen was causing the problem, and he worked with a statistician named Everett Kinsey to expand his small pilot study to eighteen more hospitals. The study results corroborated his theory, and treatment protocols were quickly adjusted throughout the nation. Patz also realized that the reason why rates of ROP were much lower in less developed countries – a fact that had puzzled many scientists – was because the incubators in those countries were more poorly constructed than those in the United States. American incubators were better sealed and fitted with holes through which gloved hands could attend to the newborn without opening the clear plastic roof. In contrast, though doctors in developing countries still pumped concentrated oxygen into the incubators of premature babies, this oxygen continuously escaped because the incubators were opened and closed several times a day to attend to the babies. This shortcoming paradoxically benefited these babies because it meant that they were effectively exposed to much lower levels of oxygen and were thus less likely to develop ROP.

Unlike Harold Ridley, who had to wait decades before seeing the benefit of his work come to light, Patz had the satisfaction of seeing the widespread reduction in high oxygen delivery result in a 60% decline in blindness from ROP in the United States within a short time.

The sight of tens of thousands of babies had been saved.

And there was little doubt about who deserved the credit for this remarkable achievement.

In 1956, at the age of thirty-six, Arnall Patz, along with Dr. Kinsey, received the Lasker Award, considered the highest honor in medicine. That same year, Jonas Salk received the award for developing the polio vaccine. At their ceremony, Helen Keller presented Patz with his award.

It would have been hard to top such an impressive start to his career, but Patz continued to make important contributions to ophthalmology. He was instrumental in the development of the argon laser as a tool to treat retinal vascular conditions. This laser became the mainstay of treatment to halt neovascularization in ROP and also from diabetic retinopathy, macular degeneration, and retinal vein occlusions. He helped organize large national clinical trials to study diabetic retinopathy and served as president of the American Academy of Ophthalmology. He rose to become the director of the

Wilmer Eye Institute at Johns Hopkins University, where he trained many future ophthalmologists and retinal surgeons who have gone on to make their own contributions to the field.

Throughout his life he was revered by the colleagues and residents who worked with him and was well-known for being friendly, patient, and kind. In every first-hand account he gave about his discovery, he downplayed his own contributions and made special effort to credit other doctors who had had similar ideas, never failing to mention how the efforts of others also helped uncover the mysteries of ROP.

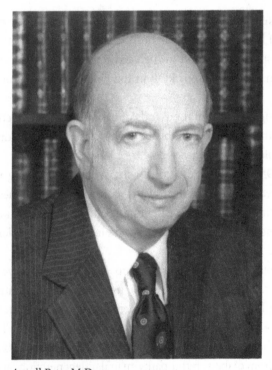

Arnall Patz, M.D.

In 2004, Patz received the Presidential Medal of Freedom, our highest civilian honor, from President George W. Bush, who called him "the man who has given to uncounted men, women and children the gift of sight." The boy from Elberton had made good. He died in 2010, at the age of 89.

———

I stayed out of the way as the anesthesiologists worked on Danny's tiny body. They got an IV started, an impressive feat in my eyes. They intubated him by threading a thin plastic tube down his pencil-thin trachea. Next to the adults, Danny looked even smaller than the dolls my twin daughters play with.

They were ready for me. I opened Danny's eyes. The pupils were still not well dilated. I don't know why I expected them to be. I looked inside the eye. Now that Danny was under anesthesia and wasn't moving, things *were* a bit easier. The vessels that emanated from his optic nerve looked dilated and sinuous, like thick rivers of sludge snaking their way across the back of the eye. There was also plenty of neovascularization and blood that blocked entire sections of my view of the peripheral areas I needed to laser.

I heaved a sigh and got started.

I applied 1,800 laser spots to the peripheral retina of the right eye, enough to fill up all the areas I could see. The problem was the areas I couldn't see well enough to treat: this was maybe 20% of the total. These untreated areas would continue to emit VEGF molecules, which could continue to promote the growth of neovascular blood vessels. I thought about treating these sections with a cryoprobe, the freezing probe that Charles Kelman had experimented with. But I would still have to treat areas that I couldn't see, which made me nervous, and I *thought* the heavy laser I'd applied in most of the periphery would be enough…I hoped it would be enough.

The left eye looked similar to the right, and I got almost 2,000 laser spots into that eye.

When I was finished I took off my headset and stretched my cramped neck and shoulders for a while. The anesthesiologists and nurses were hovering over Danny's tiny body again. I thought about what I'd have to do if Danny's retinas detached, but pushed the thought from my mind. For now, I'd done all I could.

What's ironic about the story I've related so far is the fact that I don't know a single ophthalmologist who likes treating ROP, and for over a decade, there has been a growing crisis because more and more qualified pediatric and retinal ophthalmologists will not treat and screen for the disease. There are many reasons for this, and it's worth taking some time to explain it.

For one thing, it should be acknowledged that the ROP workload is higher than it's ever been before. The rate of premature births has increased steadily, keeping pace with advances in neonatal medicine's remarkable ability to keep premature infants alive at younger and younger ages. From 1981 to 2008, the rate of premature births increased from 9.4% to 12.7%. In addition, the guidelines for ROP treatment have been periodically updated, in favor of earlier treatment, which has increased the number of treatments needed and necessitated more frequent screening of all premature infants.

But these factors actually have little to do with the real reason for the shortage of willing practitioners. What's the real reason?

Liability.

The thing that makes doctors avoid ROP like the plague is our fear of getting *sued*.

A 2006 survey by the American Academy of Ophthalmology showed that only fifty percent of pediatric and retinal ophthalmologists treated or screened for ROP, and that *twenty percent* of those who did treat were planning to stop treating within the next year. What was the most significant factor in their decision to stop treating ROP? Sixty-seven percent cited medical liability.

To understand why doctors feel this way, you have to get a sense of how the medicolegal system in our country works, and how it influences doctors' decisions every day. When I was in medical school, we were made to feel that it was not a question of *if* we would ever be sued, but a question of *when,* and *how many times,* because getting sued had little to do with being a good, smart, or ethical doctor – it was a simple matter of statistics. Simply put, statistics show that some patients don't do well. Some patients with a headache die from a brain tumor. Some patients with indigestion die from a heart attack. Some patients with ROP get retinal detachments and go blind. All of these bad things can happen even if a physician does everything he or she can to treat, support, and care for his patients appropriately. When something bad happens, we call it *maloccurrence.* There is a big difference between maloccurrence and *malpractice* – when a physician's negligence or incompetence is directly responsible for patient harm; but, in our litigious society, the distinction between these terms is too often ignored.

This is why ROP is the third rail of my field. A baby who has ROP is less likely to see well, period. Even if no laser treatment is ever needed, premature babies have higher incidence of retinal detachment, high myopia, cataract, and glaucoma, than the general population. Even when a laser treatment or surgery is performed perfectly and at the appropriate time, the retina can still detach later and the baby can go blind. The law permits a minor to sue up until he or she reaches the age of twenty, which greatly increases the liability risk of physicians who treat newborns. Some law firms even advertise specifically to patients who have a history of ROP, encouraging them to get a free consultation in the hopes that something resembling malpractice can be discovered and prosecuted.

There is nothing more distressing and emotionally taxing to a physician than being sued. There can be cases of true negligence, of course, which *should* be prosecuted. But most people know that far too many frivolous lawsuits enter our legal system, and when a physician is sued, sometimes his insurance company will recommend that he or she settle the case even if the doctor feels confident no malpractice occurred. This is because the insurance company can never predict what a jury will do. Even if the physician knows he did everything appropriately to try and save the sight of a child, when the members of a jury see a blind child, they naturally feel great compassion and sympathy. They may feel that the child's family deserves help. In the back of their minds, they might tell themselves that the doctor isn't really going to have to pay the million dollar award to the family – only his insurance company will.

And what if the doctor absolutely insists on fighting the accusation of malpractice by going to trial; and what if he wins? It is a Pyrrhic victory. Months or years of emotional distress, tens of thousands of dollars in legal fees, and the hassle of having to explain the case on every licensing form for the rest of his career – this is the price of being sued, even if the case is won. There are few negative consequences to the plaintiff or the plaintiff's lawyers, no recompense of legal fees to the defense, no reproof for bringing to the courts a long, expensive, and perhaps frivolous lawsuit. These are the reasons why an insurance company will sometimes ask the doctor to settle, why some patients with a poor outcome can feel fairly confident about getting paid, and why many lawyers continue to find medical malpractice a very lucrative field to practice in.

But why should *you* care about this? Why should *you* care if doctors are getting sued? It's not affecting you.

Or is it?

There are hidden costs to our litigious medicolegal climate. First, a doctor may not be around when you need him because the high cost of malpractice insurance is driving some doctors out of medicine. My father-in-law practiced obstetrics and gynecology. When he reached the age of sixty, after he'd been practicing for about thirty years, his annual malpractice premium was well over $100,000. Put another way, he had to deliver forty to fifty babies, or work for about four months, to cover this cost. Only then would he be able to start paying for the rest of his overhead and, after that, begin to make a profit. It's no wonder that he, like many of his colleagues, stopped delivering babies and instead chose to stay in the office doing only gynecology work. He loved delivering babies. He had more experience and expertise than his younger colleagues, but it didn't make any financial sense to keep doing OB. And as a result, in many parts of our country, finding an obstetrician to deliver your baby is a very difficult task. Similar changes have happened in fields like neurosurgery and trauma surgery.

The second reason you should feel concerned about medical malpractice is that a doctor's fear of getting sued promotes *defensive medicine,* which is a main driver of the exponentially increasing healthcare costs in our country.

Defensive medicine refers to a doctor's propensity to order tests to confirm, rule out, or document a diagnosis which he or she may already be fairly certain of, based on his or her clinical exam and judgment. In medical school, we were taught not to order a test unless the result would change the plan of treatment. In reality, doctors order tests to great excess. Let me give you the "headache" example.

You are an emergency room physician. Your patient has a bad headache. Based on your history-taking, clinical exam, and experience, you believe there is a greater than 99% chance that the patient only has a headache which will resolve on its own or be improved with ibuprofen or acetaminophen (Tylenol®). But there still may be a one-tenth of one percent chance that the patient has a brain tumor that is causing the headache and might kill the patient someday. Should you order a CT scan to make sure there's no tumor?

What would *you* do?

As the doctor, there is no incentive for you NOT to order the CT scan. There's no cost to you, and what if you don't get the test and the patient really does have a brain tumor? You can bet there would be an extremely high chance you would get sued for "missing" the tumor and not ordering a scan. You might even be a conscientious doctor who cares deeply about the exploding costs of healthcare, but you care more about your own skin, and may rationalize that the cost of one CT scan, anywhere from $1,000-$3,000, won't make much difference in the grand scheme of things. Besides, weren't we also taught as doctors to think, "What would I do if this patient were my mother?"

Of course you're going to order the CT scan.

But the problem is, ordering the test is not *cost-effective*. The chance of it being the one in several thousand who might have a serious problem is not an effective use of resources in a system with limited resources. If we keep doing things the way we've been doing them, if we keep practicing medicine like there are *unlimited* resources, healthcare will continue to bankrupt our country.

Incidentally, there are approximately 70 million CT scans performed annually in the United States. That's equivalent to one in five Americans getting scanned each year, or almost 200,000 scans performed each day.

When I examined Danny's eyes a week after his laser treatment I prepared myself for the worst. Would there be a tractional retinal detachment? Would I have to explain to his parents that I'd done everything I could, but that the prognosis for Danny to have useful vision would still be very poor?

Mom and Dad were visibly nervous. We were back in the NICU, no general anesthesia here, which meant I'd have to swaddle Danny to immobilize him. Then I numbed his eyes and put the metal speculum in to hold his lids open. This, of course, made Danny go berserk. His shrill screams, surprisingly soft because his lungs were so small, drove both parents to tears.

I took a look.

The retina was flat in the right eye. *Yes!*

There was less blood and the vessels were less tortuous. The fronds of neovascularization were almost gone. The left eye looked good, too.

It was better than I could have hoped for. I felt confident that Danny's retina would remain attached, and that the treatment had dramatically improved his chances of developing good vision in the future.

I got a hug from Mom and Dad that day. That felt good.

Arnall Patz would be disappointed to see that many ophthalmologists avoid treating retinopathy of prematurity today. I don't think he would be angry; he wasn't the type to get angry. But he might shake his head a little, and perhaps scratch it out of confusion, because the unselfish man from rural Georgia who spent his own money – no, borrowed the money – to conduct the first sight-saving study in premature infants would simply not understand the way we think today.

We don't want to treat babies because we're afraid of getting sued.

JUDAH FOLKMAN, ANGIOGENESIS, AND THE TREATMENT OF WET MACULAR DEGENERATION

"My uncle was a Nazi, but my father wasn't."

"He wasn't?" I asked.

"No, he was only Wehrmacht, just a foot soldier. He didn't talk much about it; I didn't ask."

"Did your parents come to America with you?"

"No, no. They were too old. But they were happy for me. To marry an American G.I. was a good thing, a great thing. To get out of Germany was already wonderful, to be going to America – the best."

"So life was hard after the war ended?"

My patient, Mrs. G., nodded grimly. "There wasn't enough food.

I remember not eating meat for weeks. The first time I had chocolate was when an American soldier gave it to me. It was the best thing I'd ever tasted." Mrs. G. smiled softly as she said this, as if she still held the flavor in her mouth.

"He wasn't the one you ended up marrying, was he?" I joked.

She laughed so loudly that it startled me. "No, no. I was only a little girl."

I grinned.

I liked this lady. She was seventy-eight, and her hair was almost white. Her German accent reminded me of a nice old lady who lived in my neighborhood when I was a kid.

"I was reading the newspaper on a street corner when the one I married just came up to me."

"What did he say?"

"What do you guess?"

I shrugged.

"He said, 'Do you speak English?'"

I laughed. "I bet you never finished reading that paper."

Mrs. G looked past me toward the square of light projected on the wall opposite her. Then she took off her glasses and looked at the lenses like they were broken. "That was a long time ago. Now I don't read so good."

We started to talk about why her ophthalmologist had referred her to me. She'd had dry age-related macular degeneration (AMD) but stable vision for years. Lately, she thought her left eye was getting worse.

"I see a gray spot in the middle," she said as she jabbed her thumb at her left eye. "It blocks out people's faces and the middle of words. I can't see around it." She tilted her head from side to side like a dodging boxer and peered across the room. "It's always right in the middle."

Her vision was 20/70 in the left eye. When I looked inside at her macula, I saw that it was dotted with large yellow deposits called *drusen*, the classic sign of dry AMD. There was also an irregular grayish mound right underneath her fovea, at the center of the macula, and this was surrounded by subretinal fluid and a hemorrhage that curled away from the center like a fishtail.

The eye had developed *wet* macular degeneration.

Think of wet AMD this way. There's a layer of tissue underneath the retina called the choroid. The choroid layer has tons of blood vessels, and these vessels are more porous than most, meaning proteins and serum can leak out of them more easily than they can from blood vessels in other parts of the body. There is a barrier called *Bruch's membrane* that normally separates the choroid from the retina, but sometimes, with age, the membrane breaks down. When this happens, the leaky blood vessels of the choroid can grow upward, through the degenerating barrier, and under the retina to form a complex of abnormal blood vessels called a *choroidal neovascular membrane*. This neovascular complex of vessels usually begins to leak serum and blood, and because it's happening in the macula, which subserves central vision, patients develop distortion and blurring straight ahead, at the center of whatever they're looking at.

"Tell me the truth, Doctor," Mrs. G. said when I put down my lens and pulled the slit lamp away from her. The dark vessels at her temples were pulsing. Her hands were balled into two tiny fists.

"Am I going to go blind?"

Patients ask me this question all the time. Their minds jump straight to their greatest fear: blindness. Understanding this fear helps me remember that, even though I may repeat the same explanation a dozen times a day, for each patient, it's scary, new, and possibly one of the most important conversations of their lives.

"You won't go completely blind from macular degeneration. You'll retain your peripheral vision."

She shook her head slowly and looked away. "I had a friend who got this disease. He lost his driving license. He can't even read anymore." She covered her better right eye with her hand and peered at me with her left eye wide open. "You're a blur with this eye. How did this happen to me?"

"There are two kinds of macular degeneration," I explained. "The *dry* kind is more common and usually progresses slowly. It can be stable for a long time. We call it *wet* when blood vessels under the retina leak and bleed, right in the worst possible place, the macula, which you use for central vision."

She nodded. "That's what they told my friend. Is that it? It's not going to get better?"

"If you came to me six years ago, I'd have to say you were in a tough spot. We used to do laser treatments to try and stop the bleeding, but they usually wouldn't make vision better. We used to be happy if we could just slow down the vision loss, because that was the best we could do. We couldn't bring vision back."

"You said 'used to?'"

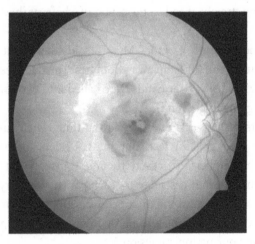

An example of wet macular degneration with hemorrhage underneath the central macula.

Courtesy of the National Eye Institute, National Institutes of Health.

"Yes, thankfully, we now have medicines that are very good at stabilizing the vision. And in about forty percent of patients, the vision actually improves. This is a lot better than anything we had before."

Mrs. G. nodded slowly. I could tell she was mulling the 40% statistic in her mind. I think she thought it sounded like pretty good odds because her worried face became more determined.

"But how does it work? I really want to know everything."

"The medicine helps stop the growth of the abnormal blood vessels. It's made up of antibodies which seek out and bind a molecule called *VEGF,* which stands for *vascular endothelial growth factor* and is important for blood vessel growth. When the antibodies bind to VEGF molecules, they inactivate them and this stops the abnormal vessels. Remember, before we got this drug most people would just keep on losing more central vision. It's is the closest thing to a miracle drug that I'll probably ever see."

Mrs. G. was silent for a while. I could hear the clock on the wall ticking slowly. I stared at her dark blue eyes and wondered for a moment what sorts of things she'd seen as a child in Germany after the war.

Then she looked at me and said, "All right, let's do it. It doesn't sound like I have much of a choice, do I?"

I'm not too young to remember what it was like before these "miracle drugs" came out. I'd spent many afternoons as a medical student standing in the corner of exam rooms, watching attendings counsel their patients for wet AMD.

"But it'll come back, right Doc?"

"I'm sorry, but your vision probably won't get any better than it is now. The important thing now is to stop the leaking blood vessels. We can laser them, but you also need to know that since the laser would damage the macula, it might actually make your vision worse...but in the long run this might be less worse than doing nothing."

Less worse?

The first time I heard these two words together I realized what a terrible burden wet AMD really was. It's one thing to go suddenly blind from an accident, or to die suddenly from a heart attack, or to be hit by a car that you never saw coming, but to live each day *knowing* your vision was going to get worse? Knowing it was practically *guaranteed* to get worse? This was like getting terminal cancer. And here was the doctor telling you you're going to die, and there's nothing he can do to stop it.

In 2000, a better way of treating abnormal vessels under the fovea became available. It employed a non-thermal laser and was called *photodynamic therapy*, but even this treatment wouldn't *improve* vision. The best outcome we could offer to patients was the hope that their vision would remain stable.

Everything changed in 2005. Genentech had manufactured a new drug called *Lucentis®*, an anti-VEGF antibody, and the one-year results were going to be presented at a big retina meeting in Montreal. I remember sitting in the audience, watching the results go up. It was incredible. There was a graph with two diverging lines, one going down gradually, showing the vision of the control patients who hadn't gotten the drug, and another line going practically straight up before plateauing. This represented the average visual improvement of the group of patients who'd gotten Lucentis. Ninety-five percent of patients on treatment retained stable vision. Forty percent had meaningful improvement in vision. A wave of excitement coursed through the audience. Doctors were gasping in surprise, murmuring in disbelief. I felt it, too. The goosebumps. The anticipation.

This was going to save the vision of millions of patients. This was going to change everything.

The story of this medical breakthrough originates with the career of one man, a young surgeon named Judah Folkman, who, forty years ago, dreamed of defeating cancer by cutting off a tumor's blood supply. At the beginning, he had no idea that his theories would make him a medical pariah for decades. And even after it became clear that his ideas had merit, he could not have dreamed that his work would one day reach far beyond the treatment of cancer, and be used to save sight.

On February 24, 1933, in Cleveland, Ohio, a rabbi named Jerome Folkman and his wife Bessie celebrated the birth of their first child. They named him Moses Judah Folkman, but he would always go by Judah. Shortly after the boy's birth, the family moved to Grand Rapids, Michigan, where Rabbi Folkman had been hired to serve the city's small Jewish population. Like most kids growing up during the Depression, Judah Folkman's childhood was frugal and austere, but his upbringing was unusually blessed by rich intellectual training under the direction of his father. Few days went by without Rabbi Folkman leading a discussion of history, religion, or science with Judah and his siblings, David and Joy. Around the dinner table, he expected each child to talk about something they had learned that day. Childish questions were entertained, and encouraged, but there was also a seriousness underlying those precious hours with his father that ingrained a sense of responsibility in Folkman. Above all, Rabbi Folkman exhorted his oldest son to, "be a credit to your people." And thus, Judah Folkman understood that he was expected to live a life of consequence.

Rabbi Folkman valued moral wisdom as much as intellectual ability, so when Folkman turned seven, he began bringing him along on his Saturday hospital visits. Folkman would watch silently as his father comforted and prayed with patients from their congregation. By this time, the rabbi already knew his oldest son had a sharp mind, and that he was not afraid of hard work. It was no secret that he aspired for the boy to also become a rabbi.

But instead, Folkman was developing a penchant for science. A biography of Isaac Newton was a favorite bedtime story. He spent hours conducting experiments with his Gilbert science set in the basement. When he was ten, he worked up the courage to tell his father that he didn't want to be a rabbi. The hospital visits had instead stirred an aspiration to become a doctor, someone who could make people better, not just console them. To Folkman's surprise his father took the news well. He merely said, "In that case you can be a rabbi-like doctor."

With his father's blessing, Folkman set his sights on getting into medical school. When the family moved to Bexley, Ohio in 1947, he began volunteering as an orderly at the Ohio State University Hospital in nearby Columbus. There he met Dr. Robert Zollinger, a well-known surgeon who invited Folkman to work in his canine lab. Dr. Zollinger was impressed by the high schooler's ability to quickly learn surgical procedures on the dogs, and Folkman proved to be a hard working, reliable asset to the lab. When it came time to apply to colleges, Folkman initially thought of the Ivy League, but Dr. Zollinger tried to convince him to stay at Ohio State so he could keep working in the lab. If Folkman stayed, Zollinger pledged to help him improve his surgery skills, so that he would arrive at medical school far ahead of his peers. Folkman did stay, and four years later he became the first Ohio State graduate ever to be accepted to Harvard Medical School.

Even before medical school began, Folkman had decided he wanted to become a surgeon. His hands were steady, his mind focused, and he loved operating – on dogs, anyway. But there was also something different about Judah Folkman. Surgeons, as a group, were not known for their intellectual curiosity. In fact, surgeons were sometimes mocked by their counterparts in internal medicine for being dense, obtuse, and even unintelligent. Surgeons also had a reputation for being aggressive and arrogant. Folkman hardly fit this mold. He wasn't a jock. He wasn't macho. And most atypical of all, he loved research as well as surgery. As a medical student, he developed one of the first pacemakers while working in the lab of Dr. Robert Gross, a well-known pediatric heart surgeon. Folkman graduated near the top of his class in 1957, and was accepted to the surgical residency at the prestigious Massachusetts General Hospital in Boston.

His surgical training was intense and almost inhumane by today's standards of residency training, which limits the work week to 80 hours. Folkman probably spent 120 hours or more per week on duty – and his residency was six years long. But he never burned out or gave up. He found time to court and marry his wife, Paula, and he loved finally being in a position to help patients. So, in 1960, he was disappointed to receive his draft notice, which meant interrupting his training to serve two years in the Navy. What he didn't know was that this hiatus from surgery would change the course of his career and initiate a four-decade long odyssey.

The Navy sent Folkman to the Naval Research Institute in Bethesda, Maryland. The post was a lucky assignment – he could have been sent overseas or put on a ship. But it was the height of the Cold War. The Russians had launched Sputnik, and the U.S. military wanted every doctor and scientist they could find to improve America's technological capacity. Folkman and a doctor named Fred Becker learned they would be working together on an assignment of the utmost importance to the Navy's new fleet of nuclear aircraft carriers. These gigantic ships were capable of operating at sea for up to a year at a time, but for one limiting factor – the shelf-life of blood. Stored whole blood lasted only a few weeks, and it was nearly impossible to keep a carrier's blood bank adequately supplied. Could Folkman and Becker help develop a blood substitute that could be stored for longer?

The two young doctors began by studying hemoglobin, the component of blood that carries oxygen to the body's tissues. They managed to dry concentrated hemoglobin into a powder form that could be reconstituted with water. But how could they test whether this "just add water" blood substitute would actually work? They decided to see if the hemoglobin solution could keep an organ alive. Folkman designed a clear plastic box that would hold a rabbit thyroid gland. He used plastic tubing to keep the hemoglobin solution running from an oxygenator, into the box, onto the organ – bathing it, and back out again to the oxygen source. Could they keep the isolated organ alive artificially?

It worked.

They were able to keep thyroid glands healthy, pink, and alive in a box for two to three weeks using just their hemoglobin solution. Becker inspected samples regularly under a microscope, confirming that the thyroid cells were definitely alive.

This success led Folkman to wonder what else they might be able to do with this thyroid set-up. Could their hemoglobin solution do more than just keep a thyroid-in-a-box alive? Would the fluid be enough to sustain new growth as well? If so, they would prove their fluid was even more analogous to actual blood and go a long way toward showing it could be useful in humans.

Folkman and Becker decided to inject some cancer cells, specifically mouse melanoma cells, into the thyroids to see if the cells would grow. They expected cancer cells to grow rapidly. Sure enough, the cells multiplied and soon the thyroids were dotted with small, pinpoint black tumors. Their blood substitute was supporting growth.

But then something peculiar happened.

After a few days, the melanoma tumors stopped growing.

All of them.

And what was more perplexing was that they were all the same small size, each only about a millimeter in diameter. This was very unusual. In real life, tumors are not all the same size. If melanoma cells had metastasized from the skin and invaded the thyroid, for example, there might be some big tumors and some small tumors, some round ones and some irregularly shaped ones.

Folkman and Becker scratched their heads. Nothing else had changed in their experiment. The hemoglobin solution was still going in, the thyroids were still alive. They presumed the melanoma cells must have died for some reason, but when they examined the cells under a microscope, they were still alive! Why had they stopped growing?

Baffled, the two doctors decided to transplant the tiny black tumors into live mice to see what would happen. The results shocked them. The tumors immediately began to grow again, becoming huge black masses. They grew so fast that the mice were all dead in short order.

What was going on? Why had the cancer cells stayed alive but dormant in the thyroid tissue-in-a-box, and then erupted into killer cancer cells when transplanted to a live animal?

The two of them looked at their samples under the microscope again and now they realized there was one obvious difference: the tiny tumors from the thyroids-in-a-box didn't have any blood vessels in them. In contrast, the tumors taken from the dead mice were completely invested with blood vessels. In a live animal, it seemed that cancer cells had somehow gotten the surrounding blood vessels to grow towards them, giving them the nourishment needed to resume growth. The thyroid samples in a box were isolated, with no nearby blood vessels to draw from. Could this be why they'd stopped growing?

Folkman knew he'd observed something important, but he wasn't sure exactly *what*. For the first time, he asked himself the question that would define his career – what would draw blood vessels toward cancer cells?

And like Harold Ridley, whose observation of inert plexiglass in Mouse Cleaver's eyes prepared him for the groundbreaking realization years later that the same material could be used for an intraocular lens, Folkman would file away this observation and have it ready when the time came.

———

"Whaddya mean it's a *shot*? In my *eye*?"

Mrs. G looked terrified.

"I know it sounds bad, but we numb your eye and it doesn't hurt. Yes, we inject the medicine in your eye. It's very fast." I might as well give her all the bad news at once, I thought. "Like I said, the medicine is very good, but one problem with it is that it doesn't last very long and the injections have to be repeated."

Her eyebrows went up. "Repeated? How many?"

"To be honest, the study that showed these medicines work did an injection every month for two years. That's twenty-four injections in two years. Now, we don't think we need to do that many, but the first three injections were the most important, so we usually start out with three in a row."

She stared at me, expressionless.

I went on, "And you need to know there are actually two medicines you can choose from. Both are made by the same company and most doctors think they are equally effective. One medicine, Lucentis, was the one they used in the study, so it's FDA-approved. The thing is, it costs $2000 per injection."

"What the hell?"

"Hold on, your insurance will pay for it."

"Really? Medicare?"

"Yes, Medicare will pay for 80% of it. I see you have co-insurance, which should cover the rest. But let me finish. There's another medicine called *Avastin®*. Like I said, it's made by the same company and works the same way. It's not FDA-approved like Lucentis is, but doctors all over the world have been using it for years, and we believe it's just as safe and effective. Plus it's a lot cheaper. It costs about $50."

"Is that all?"

"Yes. It doesn't make any difference to me which one you choose. I can tell you that I would be fine with getting Avastin if it were my own eye. It's a whole lot cheaper, but since your insurance would pay for either medicine you might not care about that – "

" – Are you kidding?" she interjected. "$50 versus $2000? For each shot? I've never wasted money in my life and if you think these two are the same, it's fine with me to go with the cheaper one. You think I want our country to keep going broke? I trust you, Doctor."

"That's fine. We can always switch medicines if you ever change your mind."

I numbed Mrs. G.'s left eye with an anesthetic gel. I used a speculum to keep her eyelids open and put in a drop of Betadine to sterilize the eye's surface. Then I used an extremely thin, thirty-gauge needle to inject 0.05 ml of Avastin through the white sclera in the bottom lateral quadrant of the eye, precisely four millimeters behind the peripheral edge of the cornea.

"That's it, you're done," I said as I removed the speculum.

"You already did it? I didn't even feel it."

"Good. Let's hope it helps."

⸺

In 1962, Judah Folkman returned to Mass General after serving two years in the Navy. He was offered the chance to serve an extra year as chief resident, a high honor, and he later became the youngest-ever Chief of Surgery at Boston Children's Hospital in 1967, at the age of thirty-four.

To any outside observer, Folkman was a shining star, a truly gifted surgeon who had already reached the pinnacle of surgical achievement at one of the world's most prestigious medical institutions. No one would doubt that his career in surgery would prove to be productive and exemplary. Everything Folkman might have wanted was now easily within his grasp: money, prestige, security, and even fame.

But he did not want these things.

Instead he chose a path that would earn the ridicule of the medical establishment and even jeopardize his position atop the surgical world. You see, he had never quite gotten those rabbits out of his mind. He sometimes pictured the way those tiny, re-implanted black melanomas had suddenly grown congested with vessels and exploded in size, quickly killing their hosts. It still perplexed him that the tumors had remained dormant in the thyroids kept alive in a box. And unlike most surgeons, who might have been happy to spend all their time in the operating room, Folkman could not ignore his passion for research. He always knew this passion might eclipse his love of surgery, but he embraced it. He couldn't just sit back and enjoy the fruits of tenure. He had to find out what made tumors grow.

So when the new professor of surgery got his own lab in 1967, he set out to answer the questions he'd first asked in 1960. As a surgeon, he'd often observed that aggressive tumors usually had large networks of blood vessels, while benign ones had little vascular supply, and he wondered, could cancer cells have some ability to draw blood vessels toward themselves? Without a ready vasculature, Folkman reasoned, tumors might only be able to grow to a certain size, limited by lack of nutrients and oxygen, plus an inability to get rid of their metabolic waste products. That might explain why the tumors had been dormant in the plastic box, where there had been no nearby blood vessels to draw from.

But this theory didn't explain *how* a tumor might induce the growth of blood vessels. The more Folkman thought about it, the more he wondered if the cancer cells were releasing some protein that signaled the blood vessels and told them what to do. Cells were known to emit signals, like hormones or growth factors, that told other cells to divide and grow, or even commit suicide and die. Why couldn't a *growth factor* be at play here?

He began calling this theory *angiogenesis,* and when he projected his idea a step further, he realized that if such a signal could be identified and opposed, then it might be possible to cut off a tumor's blood supply and halt tumor growth altogether.

It was just a theory, but it was one he would bet his career on.

He started by replicating the old rabbit thyroid experiments using dog and rat organs. He confirmed what he'd seen before, that the tumors would grow to a certain point and then stop if there was no nearby blood supply. But when he tried to publish these observations and introduce the idea of angiogenesis, he was surprised to be roundly criticized by many reviewers of the leading cancer journals. His angiogenesis theory went against the prevailing cancer research at the time. Most scientists were focused on ways to kill cancer cells, using heat, surgery, radiation, or most often, chemotherapy. The fact was that cancer itself was a poorly understood disease. Why did cancer occur? Why were some tumors aggressive and others benign? What types of treatment would be best for what types of cancer? Doctors didn't know the answers to these and many other questions, but it seemed most logical to simply kill cancer cells directly and by any way possible. The most popular drugs were actually nothing more than poisons. One of the first chemotherapeutic agents was mustard gas, first used to deadly effect in World War I, and observed in World War II to cause low white blood cell counts in its victims. If mustard gas killed rapidly dividing white blood cells, it followed that it might also kill rapidly dividing cancer cells. In Folkman's day, protocols for other chemotherapeutic "poisons" like cisplatin or vincristine were still being studied. In addition to killing cancer cells, these drugs also killed other fast-growing cells of the hair and the lining of the intestinal tract. Patients suffered greatly as their doctors experimented with dosage amounts, duration, and frequency of treatment. The bar of success was low, and easy to assess – did the drugs kill the cancer before they killed the patient?

Yet, in spite of their limited knowledge about cancer itself, other scientists were more than ready to scoff at Folkman's new ideas. No one thought blood vessels were relevant in the least. Folkman was criticized for proposing new theories without actual data to back them up. Some said his results could not be generalized and applied to humans or other animal species; and, there was a logical counter-argument to explain what he'd observed: that blood vessels grew towards tumors simply in response to the normal inflammation that developed around malignant cells, not because of any special signal emitted by the cancer.

Folkman did not realize this was only the beginning of a long battle that would go on for decades. Outside of politely-worded rejection letters, his critics snickered that Folkman was a *surgeon* who, by definition, could not possibly be a serious researcher. He should leave the real science to the Ph.D.s. Even many of his own Harvard colleagues thought he was wasting his career on a tangent that wouldn't amount to anything. Folkman, they thought, should start doing what was expected of him and spend most, if not all, of his time in the operating room, instead of the lab.

Folkman pressed on. He knew the counter-proposal that blood vessel growth occurred merely in response to local inflammation around tumors was a valid criticism. He had to admit, there was no evidence that tumors were secreting any growth factor, and all his observations of limited tumor growth had only been seen *in vitro*, in a box or petri dish, not *in vivo*, in a live animal.

He had to find a way to show the link between tumors and blood vessels in a live animal, and in addition, somehow eliminate inflammation as a confounding factor. To do this, he decided to conduct experiments in the eye. The inside of the eye was known to be an "immune-privileged" site, meaning that it was one of the few places in the body that usually tolerated the introduction of an antigen without provoking an inflammatory response. If he transplanted tumor tissue into an eye and showed tumors drawing blood vessels to themselves, he could show that inflammation wasn't the cause. Moreover, by taking tumor cells from a rabbit and injecting them into that same animal's eye, he would not have to worry about transplant rejection.

He began the new experiments. First he implanted small tumors into the anterior chamber of the eye (the space between the cornea and the lens) where the tumors would float in aqueous fluid without access to blood vessels. Just like in the Navy lab, the tumors grew to a certain point and then stopped. Then he implanted the tumors into the iris, which has plenty of blood vessels. The tumors immediately became congested with vessels and grew larger, at an exponential rate.

The success of these experiments convinced Folkman that he was on the right track and that the tumors must be releasing a signal to induce blood vessels to grow. He gave the theoretical signal a name: *tumor angiogenesis factor,* or *TAF* for short. In 1971, he published what would become a landmark article in the *New England Journal of Medicine.* In it, he wrote:

> *It has not been appreciated until the past few years that the population of tumor cells and the population of capillary endothelial cells within a neoplasm may constitute a highly integrated ecosystem...Tumor cells appear to stimulate endothelial cell proliferation.*

For the first time, he introduced the idea that inhibiting angiogenesis might lead to an effective way of treating cancer:

> *Although the evidence for these statements is still indirect and fragmentary, it seems appropriate to speculate that the inhibition of angiogenesis, i.e., anti-angiogenesis, may provide a form of cancer therapy worthy of serious exploration.*

Folkman's words would prove prescient, but at the time, his use of words like "indirect," "fragmentary," and "speculate," prompted fresh criticism and even thinly-veiled mockery from some colleagues. These scientists considered it arrogant and premature to name a growth factor that hadn't been isolated and might not even exist. Once, Folkman asked a colleague if he thought he might be giving away too much information in his lectures. Research was then, as it is now, a very competitive endeavor, and scientists were generally cautious in what they revealed for fear of their ideas being stolen. About Folkman's theory, his friend told him not to worry. "It's theftproof," he said, "No one will believe it."

Folkman and his research assistants set to work on trying to isolate TAF. Many of today's advanced techniques for identifying growth factors and other signaling molecules did not exist in the 1970s. To start with, Folkman did little more than blend-up tumors in nutrient fluid and then search the resulting soup for molecules that might have some effect on endothelial cells, the cells which constitute the lining of blood vessels. His methods of isolating proteins from the tumor-fluid included: centrifugation, gel filtration to separate molecules by size, running the fluid over starch beads which might attract some molecules more than others, digesting the proteins with enzymes, and altering the temperature, pH or nutrient bath with various chemicals. It was difficult and painstaking work, and it would go on for decades.

Meantime, some unexpected media attention made Folkman more controversial than ever. In 1972, the national press took great interest in his talk at a medical meeting in Clearwater, Florida. Science writers were hungry for any news on the mysterious disease that, because of its status as a leading killer in the U.S., had warranted a declaration of "war" by President Nixon in the previous year. The journalists saw that Folkman was proposing a completely new way of thinking about treating cancer, and they pounced on it. The day after Folkman's talk, on March 28, 1972, the front page of the *New York Times* carried an article titled: *Tests Hint Protein Is Vital to Cancers*. The article stated:

> *A Harvard surgeon said today that his research team had demonstrated in animal and test tube experiments that the growth of most cancerous tumors was dependent on a protein substance without which the tumors reverted to a dormant, harmless state.*

The surgeon, M. Judah Folkman, said the discovery could open an entirely new approach to cancer therapy – the possibility of forcing tumors into indefinite hibernation by depriving them of this substance.

The story made Folkman a brief medical celebrity. Soon his office was fielding scores of phone calls from around the world from cancer patients asking when the new treatment would become available. The attention was unexpected and in many ways, undesired. Other researchers derided Folkman as a self-serving surgeon who was trying to camouflage a lack of supporting data with public accolades and perhaps improve his chances of winning grant money through publicity. Colleagues at Harvard began sniping at him behind his back. Other surgeons started to complain that their Chief of Surgery wasn't spending enough time in the operating room. Some blamed Folkman for raising the hopes of a public desperate for a cure, when in reality the *cure* was merely an unproven theory. And perhaps at the heart of it all was the fact that Folkman's theory was an implicit criticism of those who had focused their research on killing cancer cells alone. If Folkman was right, perhaps the medical establishment was wrong.

Despite the unexpected press coverage, Folkman, like all researchers, continued to feel the stress of constantly seeking grant money to keep his lab running. He spent a significant amount of time writing and editing grant proposals, time which would have been better spent on his actual research. In 1974, Folkman's lab reached an agreement to partner with Monsanto, a private biotechnology company, which would ultimately give $23 million to angiogenesis research. Folkman and other recipients of the grant would continue to conduct research and publish with complete freedom. In return, Monsanto would get the first shot at developing any new discoveries for the marketplace. The partnership made a lot of sense, but collaborating with a private company had never been done at Harvard. Predictably, the deal, and Folkman, were widely criticized. Opponents decried the university's loss of integrity. Would Harvard now be in the back pocket of industry? Some accused Harvard of selling its soul and of "prostitution."

Folkman was as close to being a pariah as he'd ever been. One doctor said Folkman was "purifying dirt." A member of his hospital's board told him, "You're making a mockery of research here." When he applied for one particular grant, a reviewer reportedly said, "Haven't we supported Folkman long enough on this hopeless search?" Sometimes, dozens of audience members would walk out of an auditorium when Folkman came up to deliver a talk. Postdoctoral students who might otherwise have been interested in angiogenesis were advised by their mentors to steer clear of Folkman's lab at Harvard.

His reputation was swiftly unraveling.

And at Folkman's nadir, the Harvard administration dealt him a harsh ultimatum. He was informed that, as Surgeon-in-Chief of Boston Children's, he should be doing surgery full-time or he should resign the post.

It was a bitter pill to swallow, but Folkman decided he couldn't give up his research. He resigned as Chief of Surgery.

The work in the lab went on, year after year. Though still unable to isolate a specific angiogenesis factor, in 1978, Folkman and his associates were able to show that the tumor fluid they had spent years filtering and purifying *did* stimulate growth of vascular endothelial cells *in vitro*. It was a major success. This provided the best evidence yet that a growth factor *did* exist, and scientists around the world slowly began to take angiogenesis more seriously.

Another breakthrough occurred in 1983. By this time, newer, helpful lab techniques such as liquid chromatography and mass spectroscopy had been developed. Other labs had reported that heparin, normally used as an anti-clotting blood thinner, could interact with some growth factors. Folkman and two associates, Michael Klagsbrun and Yuen Shing, used heparin and finally succeeded in isolating a factor that made endothelial cells grow. This would be called *fibroblast growth factor,* or *FGF.*

They'd done it.

They'd proved there was at least one growth factor secreted by tumor cells that induced blood vessel growth. They published in *Science*, and interest in angiogenesis suddenly skyrocketed.

Now the question was, how many growth factors might there be? And were some more important than others?

There *were* others. In 1989, a scientist named Napoleone Ferrara who worked for Genentech in San Francisco, isolated a new factor called *vascular endothelial growth factor (VEGF)*. It was later discovered that Ferrara's VEGF was identical to a molecule that Harold Dvorak, a doctor working at Boston's Beth Israel Hospital, had isolated and named *vascular permeability factor*, or *VPF*; but the name, *VEGF*, stuck. VEGF would prove to be one of the most important discoveries in the history of cancer research, and its importance would extend far beyond the realm of oncology.

Meantime, Folkman was vindicated. He'd been right all along, and now postdocs from all over the world wanted to work in his lab. He was inundated with invitations to speak at medical meetings around the globe.

But what of his dream of helping people? When would this work do patients any good?

In time, the advent of gene splicing and polymerase chain reaction to amplify the production of gene products would speed the discovery of the angiogenesis inhibitors which would make Folkman's dream a reality. It became clear that blood vessel growth was a delicately mediated balance between stimulators and inhibitors. One of the first anti-angiogenic agents to be identified was *interferon alpha*, which proved to be a dramatic treatment for hemangiomas. In 1994, Folkman's lab isolated an inhibitor they named *angiostatin*. When they injected angiostatin into mice with cancer, the animals' metastatic tumors melted away. When they treated with another factor they called *endostatin*, they were shocked to find the primary tumor itself disappeared! Folkman had been hoping his treatments would limit the growth of metastatic tumors. He never suspected that some primary cancers could be completely eradicated.

The first human anti-angiogenic clinical trials began in 1999. Compared to chemotherapeutic medications, these drugs had few adverse side effects. In 2004, *bevacizumab* (a.k.a. Avastin®) became the first anti-VEGF drug to gain approval from the FDA, for the treatment of colon cancer. This best-selling drug is also currently used to treat cancer of the lung, kidney and brain.

And, Folkman hadn't guessed how great an impact his angiogenesis work would have in another field: ophthalmology. In the 1990s, Folkman had inspired a group of ophthalmologists to investigate the role of VEGF in ocular disease. These ophthalmologists, including Evangelos Gragoudas, Joan Miller, Anthony Adamis, and Patricia D'Amore at the Massachusetts Eye and Ear Infirmary, showed that retinal pigment epithelial cells underlying the retina produced VEGF *in vitro,* and that the expression of VEGF correlated with levels of neovascularization in the eye. They subsequently demonstrated that antibodies to VEGF suppressed the kind of neovascularization seen in diabetic retinopathy and macular degeneration. These studies set the stage for the development of the first anti-VEGF medication for the eye: *pegaptanib* (a.k.a. Macugen®), released in 2005, to treat wet macular degeneration. In 2006, Genentech gained FDA approval for *ranibizumab* (a.k.a. Lucentis®), and the use of its less expensive alternative, Avastin, also became widespread. By arresting the proliferation of abnormal blood vessels that form beneath the macula in wet AMD, these medicines have saved the sight of hundreds of thousands of patients around the world.

———

After three Avastin injections, performed at six-week intervals, the leaking blood vessels under Mrs. G's macula dried up. The vision in her left eye improved from 20/70 to 20/30.

She was ecstatic.

It became easier for her to read, to drive, and to see her grandchildren's faces. She thanks me every time I see her in the office, but I've told her that she really owes a debt to Dr. Folkman.

———

Judah Folkman endured decades of criticism in his quest to elucidate angiogenesis. His theories would create an entirely new branch of biomedical science and his discoveries would impact many different fields of medicine. Today, dozens of angiogenic growth factors have been identified and dozens more anti-angiogenic drugs are being studied in clinical trials. These medicines will continue to prolong the lives, and save the sight, of millions around the world.

In the last decade of his life, Folkman was widely recognized for his accomplishments. He was elected to the National Academy of Sciences, appointed to the President's Cancer Advisory Board, and honored by dozens of prestigious awards in many countries.

On January 14, 2008, Folkman was rushing to catch a flight in Denver's airport when he suddenly collapsed. He was on his way to a meeting in Vancouver, where he was scheduled to deliver yet another important keynote address. The heart attack was fatal. He was seventy-four.

Dozens of newspapers and medical journals around the world published tributes to the famous doctor. Folkman was remembered for his warmth and humility. Colleagues recalled his love of teaching and the empathetic way he cared for his patients. Dr. Larry Norton, medical director of Memorial Sloan-Kettering Cancer Center, said of Folkman, "[He] persisted in the face of great opposition, and 30 years later, it is well accepted that cancer is not just a disease of cancer cells but also of stroma and microenvironment...He opened

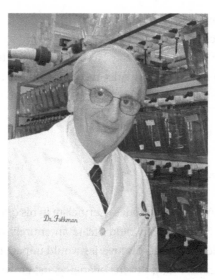

Judah Folkman, M.D.

the door wide to the impact of angiogenesis in cancer formation and treatment. And while he was recognized during his lifetime, I predict that he will receive even greater acknowledgment as we move forward."

Folkman died knowing he'd made a difference. He'd been true to his father's sacred counsel, to "be a credit to your people."

Each day, I may perform a dozen or more intraocular injections of Avastin or Lucentis, medicines that preserve and improve the sight of patients who would otherwise inexorably lose their central vision completely.

For these sight-saving treatments, we have Judah Folkman to thank.

There has been ongoing controversy regarding the use of $50-per-injection Avastin versus $2,000-per-injection Lucentis among ophthalmologists and beyond the confines of medicine. The fact is, American taxpayers, through Medicare, pay for two medicines that do the same thing, even though one costs forty times more than the other. This difference impacts Medicare to the tune of over a billion dollars each year and has galvanized those who feel cost-effectiveness should be a more important part of every medical treatment decision.

The numbers tell the story. In the United States, macular degeneration is the leading cause of blindness in people over sixty-five. 1.75 million Americans are afflicted with advanced macular degeneration, including the wet form of the disease. 9.1 million Americans have less severe, dry macular degeneration, but live in fear that they will one day develop the wet form. These figures are expected to rise to 3.8 million, and 17.8 million, respectively, over the next forty years.

In a 2008 study of Medicare patients, there were 480,025 Avastin injections (58% of total injections), and 336,898 Lucentis injections (41%). Even though the number of Avastin injections was much higher, the total cost to Medicare for Avastin was only $20.2 million, compared to $536.6 million for Lucentis.

How did this happen?

How did the *same* company, Genentech, get unlucky enough to have one of their *own* drugs become the low-cost competitor to their golden goose, Lucentis?

In Avastin, Genentech already had a full-sized antibody that would bind to VEGF and inactivate it, but they believed a *smaller* molecule would penetrate deeper into the retina, so they manufactured an antibody *fragment* to do the same thing. This was Lucentis.

Earlier in this chapter, I described the 2005 meeting in which the Lucentis study results were unveiled. I didn't mention something else I noticed, which was just as memorable as the data itself. The presenters were showing slide after slide of amazing results, each one eliciting gasps and murmurs from the hundreds of retina specialists in attendance. I looked around and noticed dozens of men in dark suits standing around the perimeter of the packed ballroom. Each was whispering into his cell phone. These guys didn't have the white and maroon-colored badges that we, the doctors, had. Theirs were green, indicating they were "non-member registrants." A few of them dashed out of the room; I could hear their voices rising excitedly once they were through the huge wooden doors. After the presentations were over, I was surprised to see an acquaintance from college among their number. He'd gone into finance and was working for a hedge fund. He, like all the green-badge guys, were professional investors who'd come to get the scoop on Lucentis.

And of course they'd come. This was going to be a billion-dollar drug. The retina community soon learned that Genentech intended to charge $2,000 per Lucentis injection. The injections were recommended monthly, so the cost of the drug would be $24,000 each year per eye; and for all we knew, the injections would need to be continued for life. I didn't know much about stocks, but I wish I'd gotten some Genentech stock before the meeting.

But then something happened that Genentech hadn't anticipated. The study results were out, but it would still be another year before the FDA approved the drug and made it available to patients. Meantime, patients were going blind from wet AMD in offices across the country. A doctor named Philip Rosenfeld at the Bascom Palmer Eye Institute in Miami decided to try injecting Avastin, the original anti-VEGF medicine which was used to treat colon cancer, into the eye. He knew that Avastin and Lucentis were both antibodies, with the same mechanism of action. He could buy the typical systemic dose of Avastin for colon cancer and divide it into dozens of smaller doses for the eye. It was a rational decision, but also a risky one.

What if this "off-label" use of Avastin caused some dangerous unforeseen effect, like stroke or heart attack? What if Avastin proved toxic to the retina? What if something else, or anything at all, went wrong? Rosenfeld could be criticized, ridiculed, and possibly sued.

At first, he only treated almost-blind patients with very severe wet AMD. The results were immediate. Just like in the Lucentis studies, leakage from the abnormal blood vessels dried up. Patients' vision stabilized, and many improved. Rosenfeld published his results and soon doctors all over the world were using Avastin. Dozens of studies soon confirmed Avastin's beneficial effect, and it appeared to be just as safe as Lucentis.

All of this was bad news for Genentech. Suddenly the legs had been cut out from under their billion-dollar drug. Many doctors did begin using Lucentis when it became available in 2006, for it could always be argued that Lucentis was *proven* to work and was safe because it had been studied more extensively and approved by the FDA; but Avastin's foothold would never be removed. Too many doctors felt it was unreasonable to pay $2,000 when a $50 medicine worked just as well, even *if* a patient's insurance would pay for the full cost of Lucentis.

Genentech began sending their sales reps into doctors' offices around the country to promote Lucentis. Then, in 2007, the company did something controversial. They announced their intention to stop supplying Avastin to the compounding pharmacies that prepared the doses for use in the eye. They claimed a fear of FDA action against them if they continued to provide the medicine to these outside facilities that repackaged it for off-label use. This decision had the potential to significantly reduce access to Avastin. Many patients without insurance or without secondary insurance would have to pay hundreds or thousands of dollars for each dose of Lucentis, if Avastin was not readily available.

Genentech's plan angered many ophthalmologists. Some of them suspected the company's decision was a calculated one, designed to increase profits. Genentech sent their president of product development to the 2007 meeting of the American Academy of Ophthalmology to defend their decision to withhold Avastin. I was there, and remember being astonished to see the normally calm and bored doctors in the audience come alive with impassioned speeches that criticized Genentech's plan and intentions. Shortly thereafter, Genentech reversed course and promised not to restrict the supply of Avastin.

The high-stakes Avastin-Lucentis battle also spilled beyond the realm of medical meetings. Articles from the *New York Times, Wall Street Journal,* and *Associated Press* carried titles like:

Genentech refuses to help study cheaper drug.

Genentech offers secret rebates for eye drug.

Genentech fights the use of its own cheaper drug.

To many, the controversy became a referendum on cost-effectiveness in medicine. Everyone thinks cost-effectiveness should be an important factor in healthcare, but in reality, it has very little practical impact on the decisions of doctors and patients. This is because patients don't actually pay for their healthcare, their insurance does. And when it comes to our own care, or the care of our families, we always want the *best* treatment, no matter the cost. This is the American mentality, and the reason why a national healthcare system will never be fully embraced in our country. But this mentality, combined with doctors' fear of getting sued and the high cost of technological advances, are the primary drivers of our skyrocketing healthcare costs.

In 2009, the federal government agreed to fund a new type of clinical trial, one meant to assess "comparative effectiveness research," and compare Avastin and Lucentis head-to-head. The *Comparison of Age-Related Macular Degeneration Treatments Trials,* a.k.a. *CATT* study, took two years to complete. The first-year results came out in May 2011.

Like all retina specialists, I anxiously anticipated the results of the CATT trial. Most of us who didn't own Roche stock, the company that took over Genentech in 2008, hoped Avastin would be found equivalent to Lucentis. If so, this would save taxpayers billions of dollars. My greatest fear was that Lucentis would be found to be superior, not by a lot, but by only a little bit. What would happen then? What if Avastin was a "9", and Lucentis was a "10"? Would Medicare be forced to continue paying $2,000 per injection to get this small additional benefit? Would our American sensibilities dictate that *everyone* should get the best medicine, no matter the cost? If so, would doctors who still used Avastin get sued? I could imagine the whole thing back-firing, with the end result that doctors would feel obligated to use Lucentis even if it was shown to be only marginally better than Avastin.

Reality was kinder than imagination. The one-year results showed that Avastin and Lucentis were equally effective. There was no statistically significant difference in visual outcome or adverse side effects. In addition, the study showed that injecting the medicine on an "as needed" basis if leakage recurred after drying up, rather than rote monthly injections, was acceptable. In 2012, the two-year results corroborated these findings.

Prior to the CATT study, many doctors felt they had to justify, to their patients and their colleagues, the use of off-label Avastin. In an editorial in the *New England Journal of Medicine,* Dr. Philip Rosenfeld wrote that the opposite was now true: "Health care providers and payers worldwide will now have to justify the cost of using ranibizumab [Lucentis]." Rosenfeld also testified before Congress in July 2011, to report that the use of Avastin over Lucentis in *one year alone,* 2008, saved Medicare $800 million dollars.

To be fair, Genentech and other biomedical companies *must* be given credit for developing sight-saving, and life-saving, treatments that benefit all of us. Without their innovation and drive, medicines like Lucentis and Avastin might not have been developed for many more years. And they *deserve* to make a profit. For every Lucentis that becomes successful, there are undoubtedly hundreds of other experimental medications that fail to prove effective, or do not make it to the market. Pharmaceutical companies investigate and develop all of these, at great expense, in the hope that one or two will become a blockbuster drug. And when they *do* hit on a winning treatment, there is no telling how long it will stay on top. New and better medicines come out all the time, and one drug's window of profitability may close abruptly. So it's easy to understand why Genentech would do everything possible to persuade ophthalmologists to choose Lucentis.

But today, more doctors than ever are using Avastin, and saving the government a lot of money by doing so. And this story is far from over. A newer drug, *aflibercept,* (a.k.a. Eylea®) became widely available in 2012. Studies have shown Eylea to be as effective as Lucentis even if dosed less frequently: every two months instead of every month. Eylea is almost as expensive as Lucentis, and it is too early to tell how much of the market it may ultimately capture. Perhaps the only certainty is that, as new medicines arrive and new studies are conducted, the treatment of wet AMD will remain dynamic and changeable.

What has *not* changed is the fundamentally flawed healthcare system we've got. Treatment decisions in medicine are rarely as black and white as in this case study of Avastin and Lucentis. Patients and doctors continue to make decisions with little regard to cost if the government or an insurance company is footing the bill.

When doctors are faced with a treatment decision, we sometimes keep it simple by asking ourselves, "What would I do if this patient was my mother?" In reality, unless we decide we want to spend even more than the 17% of GDP that we currently spend on healthcare, we may not have the luxury of adhering to this axiom. For the health of our health system, and for our nation, we might just have to use a little more common sense.

Chapter Seven | *"I really do want to see the alarm clock in the morning."*

THE EVOLUTION OF REFRACTIVE SURGERY

I was pretty nervous getting ready to perform LASIK surgery for the first time. My patient was a thirty-six year old man named Clint who sorted mail at the post office. He had a rugged appearance, with a lot of stubble on his face. I'd seen him in the resident clinic and refracted him to 20/20 vision in each eye. I prescribed him glasses. I was ready to say good-bye and move on to my next patient when he asked, "Hey, Doc. What do you think of the laser surgery?"

This is the most common cocktail party question eye doctors get asked. People are fascinated by LASIK surgery and the prospect of becoming glasses-free, but most of them don't understand how the procedure is done, and the idea of "laser" surgery scares them.

I launched into my well-rehearsed response with Clint, the same thing I repeat at least once or twice a month to a friend or relative. "Well, I think it's a very good procedure, and almost everyone I know who's had it done is very happy they did it. But you should know that there's risk to any surgery. In this case a catastrophe is very rare, but dry eye, haloes, and the chance of not seeing exactly 20/20 and still needing a weak glasses prescription are more common problems."

"Does it hurt?"

"No, it doesn't hurt. We use drops to numb your eye."

"How long does it take?"

"Not long, only a few minutes per eye, usually."

"How long does it take to heal? Do you see better right away?"

"Your eyes heal remarkably fast. You might have a little irritation in your eyes for a few hours, but many patients see pretty clearly right away. A lot of people go to work the next day."

"Really?"

"Yes."

Clint sat quietly for a while. I circled the last few items on the billing sheet and closed his chart.

"Would *you* have it done?" he asked.

"Me? Well, no," I answered truthfully. "But a lot of eye doctors would say that. We really need to see well to do our jobs, so we don't like taking unnecessary risks. I think if you want to have it done, you should make sure you go to someone who does it a lot, someone who has a lot of experience."

Clint mulled this over for a few more seconds. I was glad the morning clinic was almost over, and I was already thinking about lunch.

"Do *you* do the surgery?" Clint suddenly asked.

"What?" I said.

"Could you do my surgery?"

I sat up straighter. It was rare for a resident to come across a patient who wanted LASIK, so uncommon that it had not even occurred to me that I could be cultivating a case for myself.

"Actually, yes, I could. You'd even get a 50% discount, because I'm a resident and would have a senior doctor supervising me."

"How many have you done?"

I smiled, and almost started laughing, after what I'd just said about the importance of finding a surgeon with a lot of experience. "To be honest," I said, "I've been certified for it," which meant I'd done the procedure on a bunch of pig eyes, "but I haven't performed LASIK on a patient yet."

I thought that would be the end of it. And it wouldn't have bothered me – would I ever let someone who'd never done LASIK before touch my eyes? No way.

To my surprise, Clint said, "Well, I really like you, Doc. What would we have to do to set it up?"

Now *I* started getting nervous.

"Are you sure? Do you want to think about why you want it? You see really well with your glasses. Some people say they want it just so they can see the alarm clock in the morning, but I'm not sure that's a great reason – "

" – Actually," Clint interjected and grinned a little foolishly, "I really *do* want to see the alarm clock in the morning…and be able to go swimming and run without worrying about glasses or contacts."

He was the perfect patient. A lot of residents never get to do a LASIK case, and here Clint was, practically throwing himself at me. I swallowed hard. Everyone's got to have a first patient, I thought.

"All right…" I said hesitantly. "Why don't I bring in the senior doctor to take a look at you? We have to do some measurements, and we want to make sure you're a good candidate."

He was an excellent candidate – a mild myope, which meant he was near-sighted and could see nearby objects well, while everything in the distance was blurry. His prescription was -3.00 diopters in each eye, without significant astigmatism.

But now here I was, sitting in the LASIK suite hovering over an eye that was perfectly fine, one that could see 20/20 with glasses.

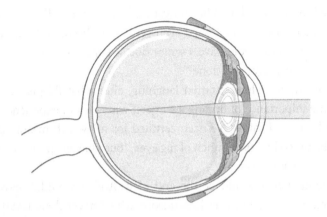

Myopia – the focal point is positioned
in front of the retina.

© 2002 American Academy of Ophthalmology

This was different from operating on an eye with a significant problem, like a cataract or retinal detachment.

Clint lay down on the table in his street clothes. I numbed his eyes with an eye drop. I sat down at the head of the table.

In myopic, near-sighted people, the light entering the eye comes to a point of focus prematurely, before it can reach the retina lining the back of the eye. This is often because the length of the eye has grown longer than normal. To see clearly, the point of focus needs to be right *on* the retina. Myopes wear glasses or contact lenses to spread incoming light rays farther apart, so that they converge at a focal point that is farther back, on the retina.

Light coming into the eye is naturally bent and focused by the cornea and the lens, but mostly by the cornea. So another way of moving the focal point back to the retina would be to *weaken* the refractive, bending power of the cornea by flattening it – by reducing the curve of its normal domed shape. In LASIK surgery, an excimer laser is used to vaporize part of the central cornea, making it thinner

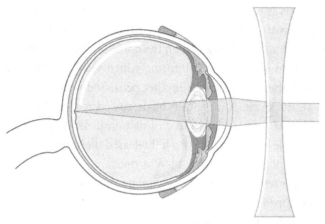

Spectacle correction of myopia – the focal point lands
on the retina, producing a clear image.

© 2002 American Academy of Ophthalmology.

and flatter. The more myopic you are, the more corneal tissue you'd
need to have zapped away. The most logical way of doing this would
be to blast away at the front surface of the cornea. This technique
is called *photorefractive keratectomy*, or *PRK*, and is still commonly
practiced today. However, PRK also ablates the cornea's superficial
epithelial cells; these cells heal back within a week or two, but in the
meantime the vision is blurry and the eye is uncomfortable.

LASIK was developed as a way to provide instantaneous
results with practically no pain. It has become the most commonly
performed refractive surgery technique. In LASIK, the surgeon
shaves a thin, hinged flap from the front surface of the cornea. The
flap is pulled back, exposing the central stromal tissue, which is
lasered, reshaping the cornea. Then the flap is flipped back into
position, perfectly covering the laser zone. *Voilá,* you're done.
The natural suction of the eye keeps the flap in place. Because the
superficial epithelial layer is intact, there's minimal to no pain and
the patient sees clearly, often right away.

I was as ready as I'd ever be. I positioned the *microkeratome,* the bladed instrument I'd need to shave the thin corneal flap, so that its suction ring was positioned on the dome of Clint's cornea. I pressed a pedal to activate a vacuum ring which would prevent the blade from slipping. I depressed another pedal and watched the machine do all the work. A razor-thin blade passed within the ring, slicing the flap of cornea like a piece of deli meat, leaving a small, uncut hinge. The blade retracted itself. I released the suction. All I'd had to do was hold it still for about ten seconds.

My attending dripped a few saline drops onto the eye. Using a blunt-tipped probe, I gently lifted the thin flap back to expose the corneal stroma underneath.

"OK, Clint," I said. "I need you to lie real still for about thirty seconds."

The laser machine projected rings and a cross-hair onto Clint's cornea to help me make sure I kept the laser positioned right in the center. It also had eye-tracking software to keep it centered even if he moved a little. All I had to do was press another pedal, and the laser started vaporizing his cornea based on the computer's pre-determined pattern. *Click, click, click, click* – what an odd sound for a laser to make, I thought. If I'd designed it I would have chosen something smoother, like a low hum. Laser spots were flying all over the field, so fast and so many that they blurred together while I stared. I thought I could make out a fine mist of vaporized corneal tissue that hung over the field for an instant, but before this thought left my mind, the laser had stopped.

The attending dripped some more saline on the eye. I used the probe to fold the corneal flap back into position.

One eye done.

I glanced at the clock on the wall. It had taken five minutes from start to finish.

I did the exact same procedure on Clint's other eye. When we were done, he sat up and blinked.

My attending said, "Clint, can you read the clock across the room? What time is it?"

Clint squinted a little, then his eyelids opened wide – he didn't have to squint. "Oh my God! I can see it! It's 4:45. This is great!"

Clint, the attending, and I gave a little cheer. Clint walked out of the office and forgot to take his glasses home with him.

—

I drove home from Clint's surgery marveling at how easy and miraculous LASIK seemed, and I immediately became curious about how it was invented. The story of refractive surgery is one of fits and starts, of abject failures, and much trial and error. It's a story that spans over a century and encompasses the work of several doctors from all over the world. Each was a risk-taking innovator who dreamed of curing one of mankind's most prevalent maladies: myopia.

The story begins, and ends, with our understanding of the cornea.

In centuries past, it is said that myopic Chinese hunters slept with sandbags on their eyes, effectively flattening their corneas to improve sight, albeit temporarily. We don't know if they understood how this sandbag trick worked – that changing the shape of the cornea altered its refractive power. It was not until the nineteenth century that we see more modern clinicians revisiting this theme. Dr. J. Ball, a physician of the mid-1800s, developed an eye cup containing a spring-loaded mallet which would impact the cornea through the eyelid, flattening it. Ball claimed the technique "restores your eyesight and renders spectacles useless." Other practitioners reportedly used a thick rubber band to accomplish a similar objective.

In 1894, Dr. William Bates, an eye doctor in New York City, did something novel. He treated a patient's astigmatism by making a corneal incision. That's right, he intentionally *cut* the cornea to change its shape. *Astigmatism* describes a cornea that has a different surface curvature in one direction compared to another. Instead of having uniform curvature in all directions, like the surface of a basketball, an astigmatic cornea is shaped like the surface of a football. A football resting on its side has a much steeper vertical curvature than it does horizontally, along the laces, and a cornea that is shaped this way produces blurry vision. Dr. Bates made a cut in the cornea that made it more spherical and dome-shaped. It was a brave, and risky, act.

We don't know if Bates truly understood why his corneal incision worked. He didn't publish more reports on it and perhaps he abandoned the technique. But he was on to something. A Dutch physician named Leendert Jan Lans is generally recognized as the first to undertake serious study of such corneal incisions, and their potential to correct astigmatism and myopia. In 1896, at the University of Leiden, he presented a doctoral thesis titled: "Experimental Studies in the Treatment of Astigmatism with Nonperforating Corneal Wounds." Experimenting on rabbits, Lans made incisions into the cornea's anterior surface and confirmed that the cornea became flatter, a change he knew would improve myopia. If he lengthened or deepened his incisions, the effect was increased. If he changed the direction of the incisions, it was possible to actually *increase* the steepness of the corneal dome centrally, which would be effective in treating hyperopia (far-sightedness). He also learned that some of the flattening effect changed over time, as the corneal incisions healed. Lans found it difficult to achieve consistent, predictable results from rabbit to rabbit, but he validated the concepts that would ultimately lead to the first successful refractive surgery technique, *radial keratotomy*, almost a century later.

Little to no work on corneal incisions was done after Lans for the next forty years. His experimental ideas were pushed to the fringe of ophthalmology and thus forgotten by many.

Fast forward to Japan, just before World War II.

In 1936, a Japanese ophthalmologist named Tsutomu Sato examined a twenty-year-old girl in his office. The patient had *keratoconus,* a disorder in which the curvature of the cornea is abnormally steep, shaped more like a mountain peak rather than the normal spherical dome. Here, the shape of the cornea is *much* more irregular than a typical case of astigmatism, and it had been impossible to improve the girl's vision using glasses. Now, Sato saw that the atypical shape of her right cornea had caused a spontaneous rupture of Descemet's membrane, which underlies the layer of endothelial cells that line the cornea's back surface. The rupture made her cornea swollen and hazy and her vision was only counting fingers. There wasn't anything to do but watch.

When her cornea healed five weeks later, Sato was surprised to find that the shape of her cornea had normalized, and that she could see much more clearly than ever before – 20/30. Sato realized that the break in Descemet's membrane had flattened the dome of the cornea, and when he thought about it more, he realized he might be able to do the same thing himself by making posterior corneal incisions.

Using rabbit eyes, Sato practiced carefully inserting a tiny blade into the anterior chamber and used it to score the back of the cornea. At first, he simply made one or two horizontal incisions in the corneal mid-periphery. When he confirmed that these incisions flattened the cornea, he began operating on patients, many of them Japanese military pilots. In time, Sato tried other incision configurations, shaped like a "T" or "V," to correct astigmatism. He also tried making incisions into the anterior surface of the cornea, but concluded that such incisions added little refractive effect compared to the posterior incisions.

In 1939, Sato published the outcomes of a series of eight keratoconus patients whose corneas had flattened after undergoing posterior corneal incisions. His successful results were celebrated in the 1940s, but over time, usually about twenty years after surgery, up to 85% percent of the corneas he had operated on became so swollen and cloudy that the corneas were ruined. By the time these complications came to light in the 1970s, Sato had died. He and other ophthalmologists of his day had not fully understood the endothelium's important role in keeping the cornea clear by constantly dehydrating it. By traumatizing the irreplaceable cells that line the back of the cornea, Sato had sentenced these eyes to a future of blindness.

The failure of Sato's techniques would mar the progress of refractive surgery for decades and produce a generation of ophthalmologists opposed to this type of incisional corneal surgery. But, across the Pacific from Japan, in Colombia, during the 1940s, a Spanish-born surgeon named Jose Barraquer had been busy inventing a totally new approach to refractive surgery. He introduced the idea of *lamellar,* meaning *layered,* surgery to alter the cornea's shape. First published in 1949, Barraquer's technique involved shaving a disk off the front surface of the cornea. Leaving the patient on the table, he'd drive the corneal button to his home workshop three kilometers away. After using liquid nitrogen to freeze the specimen, he then sculpted it into a desired new shape using a modified watch-maker's lathe. Finally, he defrosted the tissue and hurried back to the operating room, where he sewed it back into the patient's cornea. He called his technique *keratomileusis,* meaning corneal reshaping (the Greek word *smileusis* means "carving"). Barraquer later invented the first microkeratome to cut the cornea more precisely. His technique would be the precursor to the corneal flap used in modern LASIK surgery.

One day, about twenty-five years later in the mid-1970s, a Russian ophthalmologist named Svyatoslav Fyodorov was seeing patients in his Moscow office. Fyodorov had a reputation for being a surgical cowboy – he'd gotten famous by performing the first intraocular lens surgery in Russia, in 1960. His childhood had been marred by a severe injury to one of his legs after a train accident, but this hadn't stopped him from becoming a remarkably industrious and ambitious grown-up. Though the injury forced him to give up his dream of becoming a pilot, he re-directed his energy into a new passion – ophthalmology.

On that particular day, Fyodorov examined a school boy who'd been punched in the eye. A piece of glass from his shattered glasses had cut the anterior surface of his cornea. When the cornea healed, the boy no longer needed his glasses to see clearly. A small linear, off-center incision had reduced his myopia by three diopters. Fyodorov remarked, "If a fist can do this, so can I. After all, I am an eye surgeon." He knew about Sato's studies, and of his notorious complications, but Fyodorov also knew that Sato's mistake had been to incise the *back* side of the cornea. Now he thought he might be able to cure myopia by making anterior incisions alone.

For the next decade, Fyodorov dedicated himself to perfecting the technique that became known as *radial keratotomy,* or *RK.* First operating on rabbits, he experimented with corneal incisions of varying length, depth, and number. Later, in patients, he learned to arrange his incisions in a radial pattern, like the spokes of a wheel, and left a clear space in the middle which was termed the *optical zone.* Using this technique, Fyodorov achieved a high level of reliability and reproducibility.

How did it work?

Have you ever blown up a balloon and discovered that, if a part of the balloon's wall is thinner and weaker, that section tends to bulge out a little? The same phenomenon occurs when an aneurysm is formed from a bulge in the wall of a weakened blood vessel, like the aorta. In a similar way, Fyodorov's incisions weakened the structural integrity of the peripheral cornea relative to the central cornea, permitting the eye's normal intraocular pressure to make this annulus of weakened peripheral cornea bulge out. This, in turn, flattened the dome of the central cornea, reducing its refractive power and correcting myopia.

After operating on hundreds of patients, Fyodorov and his associates learned that the maximum flattening effect could be obtained with sixteen or even just eight radial incisions, not the thirty-two or even greater number they had tried in some eyes. He made his incisions deep, 90% of the depth of the cornea, to help minimize regression of corneal flattening from healing. Whereas Sato had free-handed his incisions with the naked eye, Fyodorov used a microscope and developed a pizza cutter-type tool with sixteen grooves which he used to indent the cornea and guide his incisions. He also measured the corneal thickness, something Sato wouldn't have been able to do in his day, to be more precise about incision depth; and, just to be sure, Fyodorov used a thin "dipstick" which he would place into the incisions to gauge their depth as he went along. Special instruments like super-sharp diamond blades with protective depth guards ultimately helped him make uniform incisions and reduced the risk of corneal perforation. He later developed precise nomograms to determine the best number, orientation and length of incisions to optimize the correction of different levels of myopia and astigmatism.

As Fyodorov gained confidence in RK's effectiveness, he aspired to set up clinics throughout Russia to bring it to the masses. At first, his ambitions were stifled by the totalitarian Soviet government of the 1970s; but with the ascension of Mikhail Gorbachev, whose economic reforms in the 1980s encouraged Russians to innovate and start businesses, Fyodorov's experimental new surgery was supported, and his entrepreneurial instincts were soon rewarded. He enriched himself by outfitting a medical ship that sailed to the Middle East, offering RK to wealthy clients. He set up the Moscow Research Institute of Eye Microsurgery, where he soon became famous for developing a "conveyor belt" type of operating suite in which patients on stretchers were moved from surgeon to surgeon as if moving through an assembly line. Each surgeon was responsible for only one step in the surgery, such as making one of the cuts, always the same depth and orientation, on each patient. This repetitive method was considered very successful and resulted in the most precise, reproducible outcomes. Up to 150 patients underwent RK in Fyodorov's surgical facility each day, and the waiting list grew to two years long. He also set up similar clinics in other Communist countries like Cuba. Fyodorov became one of Russia's first millionaires. He was elected to the Russian parliament, the Duma, in 1993, and he unsuccessfully ran for president of Russia in 1996.

No American ophthalmologist had ever seen radial keratotomy until, in 1976, a doctor named Leo Bores did something unusual. He went to the Soviet Union at the height of the Cold War. He wanted to see if what he'd heard about Fyodorov and his experimental surgery was true. Fyodorov welcomed him and let him observe his surgeries, examine the patients, and even operate on patients himself. Bores saw that RK seemed to work. He was intrigued, but he knew his American colleagues would still be skeptical, so he didn't tell many others about his trip when he returned home. A year later, Bores returned to Russia and re-examined the patients he'd operated on. Their eyes were stable. The patients were glasses-free. Now he felt more confident about bringing RK home to the U.S. Bores performed the first RK surgery in America in 1978. He also invited Fyodorov to the States, to give a guest lecture at the Kresge Eye Institute in Detroit.

It probably won't surprise you that there was plenty of resistance to this new, "Russian" surgery. Some of Bores' American peers accused him and other RK surgeons of needlessly operating on normal corneas to cure a condition that was not an actual disease. Others called him a "buccaneer" and ridiculed him for resurrecting Sato's failed techniques from decades earlier. Yet the buzz about RK steadily grew. The National Eye Institute initiated the "Prospective Evaluation of Radial Keratotomy" (PERK) study in 1984, to evaluate the Russian procedure. The results showed that RK was safe and effective. 65% of patients in the study no longer needed glasses. Throughout the 1980s and into the 1990s, RK was the most popular refractive surgical technique in the U.S.

So what happened to RK? Why don't we hear about people having it today?

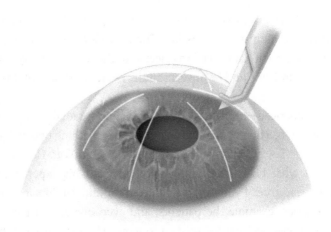

Radial keratotomy.

© 2002 American Academy of Ophthalmology.

Even at the height of its popularity, RK surgeons observed that some of their patients had progressive corneal flattening over time; some of them actually ended up far-sighted, after having had RK for being near-sighted. After a while, it became clear that the results of RK were not as stable as previously thought. RK worked, but it wasn't perfect.

The stage was now set for arrival of the excimer laser. A Russian physicist named Nikolai Basov, later winner of the Nobel Prize, invented the excimer laser in 1970. The term *excimer* derived from the terms "excited dimer." In his first prototype, Basov used an electron beam to excite a xenon dimer (Xe^2), stimulating emission of energy at a wavelength of 172 nm. This laser was a "cool" laser – it did not generate any heat and emitted energy in the ultraviolet range. Rather than burning its target material, the laser's energy disrupted molecular bonds, vaporizing it. The laser could precisely remove extremely thin layers of material without any heat or damage to adjacent structures.

In 1981, an engineer named Rangaswamy Srinivasan was using the excimer laser to cut microchips at an IBM research center in upstate New York. After that year's Thanksgiving dinner, Srinivasan wondered what the laser might do to organic tissue, so he brought some leftover turkey to his lab and tried it on turkey cartilage tissue. The result was astounding – the laser acted like a microscopic scalpel. Its energy could be precisely focused and was capable of removing tissue in incremental depths about $1/10^{th}$ the width of a strand of hair.

Srinivasan collaborated with an ophthalmologist from Columbia University named Stephen Trokel to try the laser on other tissues, like bovine corneas. By now, the excimer laser had been modified from Basov's original device, which had used xenon dimers. The newer excimer laser paired an inert gas, argon, with a halide, fluoride. In 1983, Trokel and Srinivasan identified 193 nm as the ideal wavelength to achieve maximum corneal ablation efficiency with lack of thermal injury. Each laser pulse removed precisely 0.25 microns of tissue.

In 1985, a German ophthalmologist named Theo Seiler became the first to use the excimer laser on live patients: he used it to treat astigmatism and to remove a patient's corneal scar. In 1988, Dr. Marguerite McDonald, a professor at Louisiana State University, was the first to use the laser to correct myopia. She lasered the front of her patient's cornea directly, without first creating a corneal flap. This technique was termed *photorefractive keratectomy (PRK)* and won FDA-approval in 1995.

Meanwhile, doctors had begun to combine the techniques that now comprise today's LASIK surgery: cutting a corneal flap, lifting it to expose the corneal stroma, and lasering the center of the cornea before folding the flap back into place. The method was patented by an Iranian American surgeon named Gholam Peyman in 1989; later, Greek surgeon Ioannis Pallikaris coined the term "LASIK," which stood for: *Laser in-situ keratomileusis.* LASIK became FDA-approved in 1999. Computer programs were developed to measure patients' refractive errors and calculate the optimum laser settings to correct them, greatly simplifying the surgeon's part of the procedure. Credit was given to Jose Barraquer, whose invention of lamellar corneal surgery forty years before laid the groundwork for the LASIK flap.

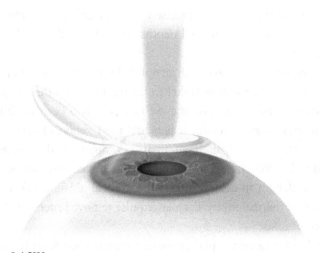

LASIK.

Today, a million Americans undergo LASIK surgery every year. The procedure is frequently used by the military to allow soldiers, pilots, and astronauts to perform their duties glasses-free. In 2010, it was estimated that over 35 million LASIK procedures had been performed worldwide, making it the most commonly performed elective surgery in recent decades. And many new advances have been developed, such as using a laser – rather than a microkeratome blade – to cut the flap, and *wavefront* technology, in which a computer creates a 3-D map of the cornea, allowing greater customization of each patient's treatment.

The collective dreams of those visionaries who sought to cure myopia have finally been realized.

———

LASIK surgery would have astonished Harold Ridley or Charles Schepens in their day. Rarely has a surgery seemed so miraculous, so futuristic. LASIK has changed the landscape of ophthalmology, not just because it can render glasses unnecessary, but also because it's changed the business of ophthalmology, reflecting new attitudes toward financial gain, self-promotion, and ethics.

The changes I'm alluding to did not emerge in a vacuum. Our healthcare system itself has changed dramatically in the last twenty years, setting the stage for a practice of medicine that is far busier and more financially-driven than in past decades. To understand the impact LASIK has had, it's important to first understand how these changes came about.

Recently, one of my childhood friends who is now a lawyer asked me, "Do you remember when everyone's parents wanted them to become doctors?" We were both Asian Americans, products of upper-middle class professional fathers with stay-at-home moms. I *did* remember thinking in those days that becoming a physician was one guaranteed way to make our parents happy and proud. I didn't know how much money doctors made, but it seemed like a lot, and even better, medicine struck me as one of those rare professions in which high compensation was coupled with the sense of fulfillment that comes from helping others. Growing up, I saw that doctors like my father, who was an interventional cardiologist, were very happy with their careers. We lived in a small city in central Illinois, and it wasn't uncommon for elderly people, whom I didn't know, to greet my dad, turn to me, and say, "Your dad saved my life. Are you going to be a great doctor like him?"

But somewhere along the path from high school to residency I noticed the world of medicine was very different from the picture I'd formed as a child. There was an increasingly obvious aura of discontent among the doctors I encountered and learned from. First and foremost, doctors complained about steadily declining reimbursement for their services. They griped about having to work harder for the same amount of income, their squabbles with insurance companies, and rising malpractice costs. A lot of them said they wouldn't recommend medicine as a career to their kids. What was going on? I couldn't understand why they were so pessimistic about a profession I'd grown up believing was among the best I could aspire to.

What I didn't know then was that the doctors practicing at the time of my youth were being extremely well paid for their services. It was the "golden age" of medicine, before managed care and HMOs, in which physicians set their own fee schedules and were generously reimbursed by insurance companies. No wonder doctors of the 1980s were a happy lot. They were raking it in.

But the old system of reimbursement was unsustainable. The pendulum swung the other way, resoundingly so. Since the early 1990's, physicians have gotten paid less and less for their work as Medicare, Medicaid, and private insurance companies have steadily cut reimbursement. Here's an example. The exact amounts varied from state to state, but in 1980, Medicare paid ophthalmologists around $2,000 to perform a cataract surgery. By 2008, this had been reduced to approximately $626; and, in addition to the operation, this fee was supposed to cover the costs of all the post-operative visits as well. Adjusted for inflation, this represents an 88% decline in compensation.

Who would be crazy enough to enter a field in which income declined by 88% over a couple of decades?

Cuts in other medical specialties have also been dramatic. In 1980, my father might have been paid $600 to perform a diagnostic cardiac catheterization – threading a thin catheter up into the heart and injecting a dye to image the coronary arteries.

Today, this procedure, which carries significant risk of heart attack, stroke, and even death, earns him $250. Every field of medicine has experienced similar declines. And every year, Medicare threatens ever larger cuts to physician pay, sometimes as much as twenty-five or thirty percent. Usually Congress repeals these large cuts at the eleventh hour because they know cuts this deep would preclude many doctors from even accepting Medicare patients. Instead, the declining fortune of physicians remains gradual...and inexorable.

So you can see why an older doctor might have become disgruntled, constantly feeling his livelihood has been under attack. For the last twenty years he has been paid less and less to perform the same services. If he wanted to maintain his current level of income he had to see more patients or do more surgeries to get it. His natural response was to do just this, by filling up his schedule and forcing himself to see more patients, faster. Early in his career he might have allotted thirty minutes, or even forty-five minutes, to evaluate a patient; now he's got only ten or fifteen minutes per patient visit. In the past he could be confident that he would be paid for his services, but now, it isn't uncommon for him or his staff to spend hours every week fighting insurance companies who refuse to pay because the proper sequence of referrals hadn't been received or because there wasn't enough time to obtain *prior authorization* before performing an urgently needed treatment. These changes have made doctors more stressed, less happy, and very likely to spend a lot of time thinking of ways to keep their income up, fighting against the tides of change.

This is the backdrop for the story of how LASIK has changed the practice of ophthalmology. First introduced in the 1990s, LASIK is an *elective* procedure. This means it isn't considered *medically necessary;* after all, these patients can generally see 20/20 with glasses. This doesn't mean that LASIK isn't a good procedure; it is, and it does provide a functional benefit. Still, this idea of "elective" surgery was new in ophthalmology. These patients didn't need treatment to prevent blindness or combat a disease, and for a LASIK surgeon to be successful, he or she would have to drum up business by finding new and willing patients...*and* compete with fellow ophthalmologists to get them.

It's easy to see why Arnall Patz or Judah Folkman might have found these realities distasteful, but in an environment of declining reimbursements, LASIK seemed to arrive at just the right time. Refractive surgery was not covered by insurance, so patients paid the typical $5,000 fee (for both eyes) out of pocket – no need to deal with insurance companies. Twenty-five percent of Americans were myopic, so the gold rush was on. Leo Bores, who had brought RK to America, put it bluntly when he wrote critically about the new refractive laser treatments: "Just feed the patient's refraction into the computer, aim the laser, push the button, and the money rolls in. Gadzooks! What a neat way to recover the lost revenue from the reduction in cataract fees!"

LASIK surgeons quickly learned to market themselves and improve their salesmanship skills. Thirty years ago, physicians would have been horrified to see another physician advertising directly to patients with billboards, print ads, radio spots, or television commercials. Such self-promotion was not only frowned upon, it was considered unethical and might have even put one's medical licensure in jeopardy. Today, advertising for LASIK has become the norm. Ophthalmologists offer free consultations, limited-time discounts, and no-interest financing to entice patients into their offices. Successful refractive surgeons learned to block off specific days to see *only* young, healthy LASIK patients, who might otherwise be turned off by sitting in a waiting room with elderly cataract patients or others with serious medical problems like corneal ulcers. The surgeon might have also learned the importance of having a modern-looking office with trendy furniture, hiring young and attractive staff people, allotting plenty of time for each patient consultation (30 to 45 minutes), and making sure to minimize wait times...all to make a more positive impression on potential LASIK patients.

How has *my* practice been affected by the changes I've described?

I used to think that when I'd "made it" and became a surgeon, I'd enjoy taking my time with each patient, learning about his or her family and past experiences. I quickly learned it's not like that at all. Sometimes I'm scheduled to see patients every five minutes. Each day is a struggle to stay close to on time, while trying to do everything for every patient to save their sight. I've become a small business owner and have realized that, to keep my business going, I've got to produce more, because the income for the service I provide keeps declining. Perhaps the most distressing impact of this new status quo is the fact that the "old-fashioned" doctor-patient relationship is a thing of the past and will probably never return. Today our healthcare system encourages patients to see doctors merely as technicians. One is probably as good as another, and as long as the co-pay is low and the wait is under an hour, it doesn't matter who's treating you.

But the good news is that I don't think the doctors of my generation are unhappy at all. Unlike older physicians, we never knew the "good old days." After a decade of preparing to enter this "diminished" field of medicine, perhaps our attitudes have been suitably adjusted. We'll never see the levels of income enjoyed by the generation that preceded us, but if making money had been our primary goal in life, we could have gone to Wall Street like a lot of our college friends did. Looking at our current economy and seeing the struggles of everyday Americans through the eyes of our patients, it's hard to complain that we aren't paid enough.

There will always be some who argue that, considering the 7-14 years of post-college training, the accumulation of hundreds of thousands of dollars in student debt, and the mental and emotional stress that accompanies our daily decisions, doctors should always be among the highest paid professionals in our society; and, that it's in our national interest to continue recruiting the best and the brightest into medicine. I acknowledge this sentiment, yet I also must admit that I would continue to enjoy my job each day even if I were paid far less. We get to *help* people. I know most doctors, when we stop to think about it, realize how lucky we are to be able to do this for a living. Sure, it's important to earn enough money to provide for your family, send your kids to college, and pay down the mortgage. But after that, perhaps the value of working for one's own fulfillment begins to exceed the value derived from working for additional money.

I think this sense of fulfillment is part of a doctor's compensation. I value fulfillment. It's worth a lot to me.

Chapter Eight | *"If I cannot discover a way to read and write…I shall kill myself."*

LOUIS BRAILLE AND NIGHTWRITING

I used to think I was pretty good at delivering bad news to patients. I'd certainly gotten plenty of practice as an intern, during that ridiculously busy year, right after medical school, when I was usually the doctor who had the closest contact with patients and their families. Here's how I might break the news:

"Unfortunately, your father suffered a very severe heart attack. We immediately gave him medicines to try and make it easier for his heart to pump blood, but his heart began to beat irregularly. We shocked his heart several times to help it return to normal rhythm, but we didn't succeed because the damage was too severe, and his heart actually stopped beating. Then we worked for almost an hour to try and restart it, but we weren't able to. I'm very sorry, but he passed away a few minutes ago."

Sometimes I had to tell patients they had cancer, or discuss whether a family should withdraw life support because a patient was not going to recover. After a while, I realized that being patient and sincerely empathetic were more important than any words I might say, but that talking a lot seemed to make *me* feel better. I had these types of conversations so often that when I started my ophthalmology residency the next year I really didn't think I'd ever be fazed by having to deliver bad news. After all, from now on it would just be working on the eye, right? Eye problems were never a matter of life and death, I remember thinking.

But then I had to tell a patient he was going to be blind. Forever.

When a patient is diagnosed with a life-threatening disease, the expectations of the patient and the family are immediately adjusted. Everyone instinctively understands that death, however much we hate to think about it, is inevitable. It's common to reflect on a life well-lived, or to consider "what's really important." Death is something we all have to prepare for.

In contrast, few people will ever be blind. When a patient becomes blind, often the rest of his or her body is doing just fine. There's no reason to believe the patient won't live for many more years, often decades. But it's the very fact that the patient is otherwise healthy, and expects to live a normal life, that makes blindness so terrifying.

And that's why, for the first time, I was completely lost when I had to tell a sixty-five year old man and his family that a *central retinal artery occlusion* (think of this as a stroke to the eye), and the *neovascular glaucoma* that succeeded it, had permanently robbed him of the sight in his right eye. Unfortunately, this particular patient had lost vision in his left eye from a childhood injury. I managed to say the words, but to me, they sounded robotic and unfeeling.

In my subspecialty of retinal diseases, I probably deal with blinding diseases more often than most eye doctors. Patients can go blind from a variety of problems: trauma, glaucoma, retinal detachment, vascular occlusions, or surgical complications. With more practice, I learned to avoid saying the terrible word, "blind." Instead, I might say something like, "I'm very sorry, but I don't think this will be a seeing eye anymore." On paper it looks pathetic, like something my kids might say, but I've realized there's really no good way to mitigate the news. You're either blind or you aren't. There's nothing I or anyone can do to bring the vision back. When you're there, in the moment, there's no distracting the patient from the dire reality by jabbering on about what was tried or how there might be a slim chance of recovery with another treatment.

Patients respond to the news in a number of ways. Many of them cry. Some get angry, at me or at God. A lot of patients become depressed.

So ophthalmologists hate blindness. It represents failure and displays our inability to help, to fix, to heal. And the most heart-rending cases are those of blind children, who were perhaps unlucky enough to have had severe retinopathy of prematurity or congenital glaucoma. You can't help but think about how limited a blind child's future will be. You can't help but pity the parents who may have to support the child into their old age. These are the times when life seems the most unfair, and when we physicians feel the most helpless.

There was one man, of course, who did more than anyone to help the blind. Everyone knows his name, but few seem to know his story. Anyone would have forgiven Louis Braille for thinking life was unfair, but for those who suspect God does things for a reason, it isn't hard to see His plan for Braille's life. For no life could better exemplify the words of the apostle John, who wrote, "As [Jesus] went along, he saw a man blind from birth. His disciples asked him, "Rabbi, who sinned, this man or his parents, that he was born blind?"

"Neither this man nor his parents sinned," said Jesus, "but this happened so that the work of God might be displayed in his life." John 9:1-3.

—

Paris 1821

There was something different about the way Gabriel was walking ahead of him in line. The thick, scratchy rope in Louis' right hand was going slack, when the line of blind boys almost always kept it taut as they pulled each other along the Champs-Elysees. They were slowing down.

What's wrong? Louis wondered.

Up ahead, Dr. Pignier's heavy boot steps were loud and familiar, a reassuring sign, but then the line almost slowed to a stop and Louis bumped into Gabriel's back.

Then he heard the trouble up ahead.

"Blindy! Blindy! See my ice cream cone? Over here!"

To Louis' surprise, it was a girl's voice, high-pitched, almost a squeal. Louis hung his head and shifted uncomfortably.

"Madam," he heard Dr. Pignier's dignified voice. "Please inform your daughter that these boys are students of the Royal Institute for Blind Youth. They are serious students and are learning to help themselves. At our school they attend classes and learn to produce useful crafts like slippers, garments, and – "

" – Shut it, old man," a woman's sneering voice intruded. "You can help these boys all you like, but there's no changin' what they're gonna be. Beggars. Every last one of 'em. Whole city's already teeming with 'em. Blind old soldier on every street corner, botherin' decent people. It's shameful. So don't you preach to us. Francesca! You get back here!"

Louis heard the woman scurry off after her daughter.

Dr. Pignier prodded the boys along and Louis felt the rope tug. He walked forward. He heard the school director's steps slow and fall back; he was drawing near to Louis in the middle of the line.

"Doctor Pignier?" Louis half-whispered, not wanting the other boys to hear.

"Yes, Louis?"

"Is it true what she said? I know there are a lot of blind beggars... what *will* happen to us when we're too old for the Institute?"

The director's voice was deep and reassuring. "My dear boy. You're only twelve. You needn't worry about such things." He sighed. "Everyone's in a foul mood these days. It's been this way for years, after all the defeats and the government going back and forth. Everyone's fed up with it."

Louis nodded, wanting to show that he understood such important matters.

"She shouldn't insult the maimed soldiers, though. Don't forget Louis, they fought for what they believed was right for France. They sacrificed for all of us. They shouldn't be ridiculed."

"But what more can they be, besides beggars?" Gabriel Gauthier called back over his shoulder. Louis' best friend, Gabriel, had apparently heard everything. "I mean, they can't *do* anything. We're learning to sew slippers and scarves. We learn to play the piano and violin. But they're grown men. They won't want to learn anything new."

"I don't know, boys, I don't know."

And Louis felt a surge of pity for the hundreds, perhaps thousands, of Paris' blind, homeless beggars. He knew some of them humiliated themselves by wearing fake donkey ears or cowbells to get a laugh, and a franc, from passers-by. He felt so lucky to be a student at the Institute, the only school for the blind in all of France, perhaps all of Europe as far as he knew. At least the school gave him a chance to learn a useful skill that might be a means of supporting himself. He was quick at sewing and stitching, maybe even the fastest boy of all, but it was his fantastic memory that he took guilty pride in. Listening closely, he could recite lessons back to the teachers word for word. How he loved to learn about history and literature! How he yearned for the chance to read books! But there was a limit to what the blind could do, and what they could become. Louis had to learn to accept that.

He smelled the familiar aroma of freshly baked baguettes. They were near the botanical garden now, though he had no memory of what trees and flowers actually looked like. He turned his head toward the snappish sound of fluttering flags – the wind was picking up, and he used his free hand to turn up the collar of his thick woolen uniform coat. The gravelly walkway was thick with the sounds of strangers' footsteps, hurrying this way and that, rustling the fallen leaves underfoot.

"It's a cloudy day, my boys," Dr. Pignier said. "A month more and there will be snow on this ground. It looks like there might be a dark cloud to the south of us." Louis smiled, thankful for the kind director. He was always so conscientious about describing their surroundings.

"Shall we rush home to open the windows? To let the rain wash out the cobwebs?" Gabriel quipped. Louis and the other boys laughed.

Dr. Pignier chuckled. "Quite an idea, Gabriel. It would be worth trying, if I wasn't worried that the shutters might fall off if you tried to move them."

The boys laughed some more. They could joke about their dilapidated building with the director, but not with the other teachers. Most of the Institute's instructors were strict and humorless, not like Dr. Pignier.

"Let's walk through the garden now, and then turn back toward home before the rain comes. It will soon be time for our history and geography lesson. Oh my, there is a fast-flying bluebird above us. He just alighted on a branch and is staring at us. Don't stare back my boys, you may scare it."

Louis smiled and shuffled along.

Louis never got used to the classroom's stale air – moldy and oppressive. He longed for the open fields of home, near the village of Coupvray. In Paris' winter the boys froze, in summer they baked – that was life at the Institute. But for the thirty minutes Dr. Pignier lectured on history, Louis forgot about physical comforts and listened, enthralled.

"Now you must understand, boys, Marshal Ney believed he could carry the field, just as he'd done a dozen times before. The cavalry charge went forward, but this time they were foiled by the enemy's square formations. His men could not break up the squares. Yes, Gabriel?"

Louis heard Gabriel's hand come back down to his desk with a soft thump.

"Were the squares like a phalanx? I mean, shouldn't Napoleon have seen they would be a strong defense?"

Dr. Pignier emitted a soft snort, a habit of his when he was pleased with one of their observations. "Quite so, the phalanx is a good analogy. If you've ever read – "

The director stopped, failing to catch himself before he'd uttered the word. He recovered quickly.

"Ahem. At any rate, the attack failed. Ney had to retreat. And – now this is controversial – he did not spike the enemy cannons as he could have. He and Napoleon would later regret this."

Louis raised his hand.

"Yes, Louis?"

"The Battle of Waterloo was lost. Marshal Ney was later executed by our own government. Should we consider him a hero or a traitor, Sir?"

There was a long silence, broken by the occasional sound of boys' feet scuffing the wood-paneled floor. The director's footsteps advanced down the aisle and stopped beside him. Louis felt Dr. Pignier's hand rest on his shoulder.

"Well Louis, politics is tricky. I've seen our government change many times, and it may yet change again. It is not for me to say whether the Marshal was right or wrong. But he did what he believed was right, of that I'm sure. At his execution he refused to be blindfolded and he, himself, gave the order to fire."

Several boys gasped. *What a sight that must have been,* Louis thought with wonderment. And he shivered at the thought of seeing a dozen rifles pointed at his heart, aimed to kill.

"Ah, my boys, let us not dwell on these sad matters. In fact, I think now is an excellent time to tell you that we will have a special guest this afternoon."

The students murmured with surprise.

"Who is it?" one boy asked.

"Ah, I think I will let you discover this for yourselves."

There was a collective moan.

Dr. Pignier laughed. "Be patient, boys. You will see, you will see."

Louis stood before the large pedestal and ran his fingers over the embossed letters in the huge book that lay open before him. He'd already read this book, *Morning and Evening Prayer,* two dozen times before, but it was still so difficult to get through. A year ago, his heart had leapt at the news he would be introduced to the school's "library." Then he learned the library contained only three books. *Only three!* His disappointment deepened when he discovered how difficult the embossed letters were to read. Decades ago, the founder of the school, Valentin Haüy, had invented the embossing system in which letters were impressed into heavy sheets of paper. The blind could then trace the raised letters with their fingertips. But the letters were hard to distinguish from each another, particularly "O" and "Q," or "I" and "T." Sometimes identifying the letters took Louis so long that he forgot what the first words of a sentence were, and he had to start over. Another problem was that the books were huge – this short book filled eight heavy volumes; each page might only hold eight or ten words. Louis returned to the books again and again to improve his accuracy and speed, but he still had difficulty. He berated himself for being too slow, too stupid – but he knew this wasn't true. Most considered him the brightest student in the school; many of the other boys had given up on reading completely. Sometimes Louis stood at the pedestal and cried quietly to himself. It didn't matter if there were others in the room; the blind boys couldn't see each other cry.

The door to the library swung open and Louis clamped his hand down on the pages to keep them from fluttering.

"Louis? Are you in here?"

"Yes, Gabriel."

"It's time for the visitor. You should come now; everyone else is already heading down."

"Alright." Louis sighed and closed the book. He felt for the wall and walked toward the door. After two years, he had every inch of the school committed to memory, but out of habit he subconsciously counted the steps: *ten steps to the door, twenty to the stairs, thirteen stairs. Turn right toward the classroom door, ten steps, the door on the right.*

When Louis entered the room he felt something was different. It was so quiet. The normal chatter and giggles of boys aged six to sixteen was absent. *Were they the first to arrive? No, Gabriel had made it sound like they were late.* Louis felt the familiar row of desks and yes, most of the boys were already here. He and Gabriel sat near the back. And then he noticed the visitor's smell. It wasn't Dr. Pignier or one of the other teachers. This man smelled of the outdoors, like a pile of wet, fallen leaves in autumn, mixed with the musky smell of a damp wool coat that hadn't fully dried. The man's odor came from behind Louis, and he tried to picture the man standing in the back, watching the blind boys feel their way to their seats.

Dr. Pignier cleared his throat at the front of the room.

"Boys, we have an illustrious guest today. His name is Captain Barbier. He is a retired captain of the artillery."

There was a murmur of surprise and excitement among the students.

Louis was intrigued. He loved military history. *Had this captain been at the Battle of Waterloo? Was he one of the lucky few to survive the Russian campaign?*

"Captain Barbier has something very interesting to share with us. But I will let him tell you all about it."

Louis felt the musk-smelling man brush by his desk. By the sound of his footfalls he was stocky and heavy, yet he moved quickly and with agility. This was one veteran who hadn't been maimed.

The captain's voice was deep and rasping. "Young men, I have come to show you an invention of mine. I hope it may be of some use to you."

The captain began to pace back and forth at the front of the room.

"You see, when I was in the army I spent some time in the Signal Corps, and one of my assignments was to invent a way of communicating on the battlefield...at night."

Louis sat up a little straighter.

"I called it *nightwriting*. I used a sharp-pointed stylus to punch dots and dashes into paper, which you can feel with your fingertips when you turn the paper over. Each combination of dots and dashes represented a sound, and the sounds put together formed orders like "attack" or "retreat." This way, we could communicate with our frontline troops at night without speaking or lighting candles that might have given away our position. It worked quite well, and I have recently realized that my method may be of some use to the blind...to you."

Louis felt an unfamiliar sensation. *Dots? Dashes?* It was like a code, a completely new idea. *What was this feeling?* It swelled up from his chest and he felt his face turn up in a broad smile. He felt giddy with delight. *This is it!* He knew almost at once that this idea could change his life.

The captain passed out a few papers with the dots and dashes poked into them.

"Because the dots and dashes represent sounds," he heard the captain say, "I've sometimes called my method *sonography.*"

Gabriel passed Louis one of the pieces of paper. Louis felt its surface. There were tiny raised dots, no bigger than pinpricks, but spaced apart so that he could clearly distinguish each one individually. He ran his fingers across the page and felt his skin rumble over a whole series of them. The sensation sent a tingle of excitement up his arm.

The other boys felt it too. They were voicing their surprise and excitement, and as more and more boys felt the pages, the previously silent room began to fill with noise.

"It's so easy to feel!"

"The page is so light! This is just like a page from a real book."

"What does this say?"

Captain Barbier laughed. "Give it a little time, young men. I will decode it for you. But first let me show you how to write with this system."

Write? Louis hadn't even dared to think of this. *Of course! Write!* Captain Barbier passed around a slate with horizontal grooves, over which paper could be positioned and a stylus could be used to poke holes into the paper. He went around the room, demonstrating different messages and showing the boys how to read them.

They spent hours in the classroom that afternoon. Many of the other teachers remained strangely quiet. Louis heard one voice an objection that the system was based on sounds, not the alphabet. Another made a disapproving comment about a system that only the blind could use, and not sighted people.

Finally, the group adjourned at dinner time. Louis' heart was still racing. He didn't want to leave. He couldn't wait to keep practicing the system. He could already see where the captain's method could be improved and made easier to use.

And he was sure he could be the one to do it.

—

Louis Braille, born on January 4, 1809, had grown up about twenty-five miles east of Paris, in the small village of Coupvray. His father, Simon René, was a skilled leather craftsman who was known throughout the region for making excellent saddles and harnesses. As a toddler, Braille spent hours watching his father work in his shop, which was filled with hanging rawhides, the smell of leather, and dozens of tools. The tools fascinated the young boy.

One day, when Braille was three years old, his father walked outside to talk to a customer and left him alone in the shop. We cannot be absolutely certain of what happened next. Many authors have considered the circumstances of Braille's injury, and presume the young boy probably climbed upon his father's chair and then onto the workbench. We *do* know that he grasped a sharp tool, probably an awl – a sharp-pointed instrument used to punch holes in leather.

It is easy to imagine the inquisitive boy grasping the awl and imitating his father by trying to make holes in a thick piece of leather. Perhaps he bent down low, to be precise about it, like his father. Perhaps he found the material surprisingly tough, and determined to stab down with all his might. And, as the most commonly related story goes, perhaps the awl slipped off the smooth leather and plunged into his eye.

What is certain is that Braille punctured his left eye with a sharp instrument. His screams would have brought his mother, Monique, and his older siblings, Catherine, Marie, and Simon, running from the house. When they burst into the workshop, they would have found Simon René cradling his son, shouting for them to bring the doctor.

But there were no doctors in Coupvray in 1812. All the doctors in the area had been drafted into Napoleon's army. Monique brought a village woman who mixed poultices. She smeared her pasty herb mixture over the eye and told them to wait and see. Eventually, a man who called himself a doctor did come and examined the injured eye. He advised the Brailles to cover the eye with cold compresses and keep their son in absolute darkness. Louis Braille stayed in his room with the windows shuttered for weeks.

In time, Braille's right eye also became inflamed. His parents believed he had transferred an infection from his injured eye to this eye, because he incessantly rubbed both eyes. Today, we believe that most likely he actually developed *sympathetic ophthalmia,* a rare condition in which the body's immune system attacks the fellow eye after a traumatic injury. To his parent's horror, his right cornea began to cloud and the eye began to lose vision. Within a year's time, Braille was completely blind in both eyes.

His world was now blackness. At first, he didn't move anywhere without being escorted by a family member. Each morning he lay in bed until someone came to get him. He rarely left the house. Slowly, he learned to move about the home, feeling his way down the stairs, along the tables and chairs. His father built him a cane that he tapped before him as he walked, learning to avoid obstacles and listening for the echoes when the sound of his tapping bounced off nearby walls. He counted exactly how many steps separated the house from the well, from the garden, from his father's workshop. Eventually, he learned to venture beyond his family property and into the village.

The people of Coupvray treated Braille kindly, for he was always cheerful and friendly, and his father was a well-respected craftsman. Braille was tall for his age, with curly blond hair. He spent hours in the village square saying hello to people and listening to other children play.

One man took a special interest in the boy, Father Jacques Palluy, the village priest. He saw that Braille was intelligent and curious, so he offered to teach him lessons. A few afternoons each week, Father Palluy read Braille stories and taught him religion and science. He gave his eager student detailed descriptions of the natural world. On their walks through the countryside Louis learned to identify the smell and feel of different flowers, and the sounds of birds and other animals. The more time Father Palluy spent with the young boy, the more convinced he became that Louis had a brilliant mind. One day, the priest proposed something unexpected.

He asked Louis if he would like to go to school.

No one had ever heard of a blind boy being admitted to the village school. In those days, the blind were generally considered stupid and incapable of learning. Many blind children were simply abandoned, and almost all blind people ended up as beggars. But Father Palluy felt confident Braille could succeed. He would ask the school master if Louis could join the class.

The school master said yes.

Thereafter, one of Louis Braille's classmates would come to his home each day to walk him to school. In the classroom, he learned to listen carefully to every word the teacher spoke, so that he could repeat the lessons verbatim. When he was asked a question, he responded quickly and correctly, greatly impressing the school master and his classmates. But when the other children worked on reading and writing, Louis sat silently, listening to the scratching of chalk on slateboards or the sound of pages being turned. He desperately wanted to read, but he knew this was impossible, and he already knew how lucky he was just to be a student at the school.

Two years later, Father Palluy changed Louis Braille's life again.

The priest had heard of a special school in Paris – a school for the *blind!* The boys at the Royal Institute for Blind Youth learned to do useful work, like sewing and knitting. They were also taught to play instruments, like the piano and violin. Best of all, they learned to *read!*

How could they read? the Brailles wondered.

The students used their fingers to feel the impressions made by embossed letters on thick paper.

Simon René worried about the tuition, and feared they could

not afford the expense, but Father Palluy said he could arrange for a scholarship.

And so, on February 15, 1819, Braille and his father departed Coupvray on the four-hour stagecoach trip to Paris. At ten years old, he would be the youngest of the sixty students at the school.

Louis Braille would spend most of his life living at the Royal Institute for Blind Youth. After his introduction to Captain Barbier's system of nightwriting, he felt sure that a method of dots would be much better than the clumsy embossing system. The captain's dot method had several drawbacks, however. First, his entire system was based on sounds, which were difficult for readers to reliably translate into words. This might work fine in the Army, when only a limited number of messages were needed, but to convey all the words and meanings of the French language? Sonography just wasn't practical.

Also, there seemed to be too many dots. Barbier had arranged for each sound to be represented by a "cell" with twelve spaces for dashes or dots, arranged in two vertical columns of six spaces. This was too many spaces. It might take over a hundred dots to form a single word; the sheer number of possible combinations was staggering. The captain's system also lacked punctuation and a way of communicating numbers. Furthermore, Braille found it difficult to make the dashes consistently using the stylus; any lack of uniformity would only make it harder for the reader.

For two years, Braille spent every spare moment punching dots into paper, experimenting, trying to improve the dot code. His classmates became accustomed to falling asleep to the sound of Braille punching holes while in bed. In time, he realized that it would be better if the dots represented letters instead of sounds. Spelling out the letters of a word would be much easier than trying to combine a word's sounds. He also did away with the dashes and decreased the number of dots by creating a cell composed of six dots, arranged in two columns of three. This cell was small enough to be entirely felt beneath the tip of one finger. Fewer dots made reading and writing much faster, and there were still enough combinations for all the letters and numbers, punctuation, and even mathematical notations.

Braille divided the alphabet systematically, into thirds. He devised simple combinations using only the top four dots to represent the first ten letters of the alphabet: A through J. Then he simply added the bottom, lower left corner dot to the first ten combinations for the letters K through T. The final bottom right dot was used for the remaining letters, U through Z. It was simple and easy to learn. It was ingenious.

In 1824, Braille was ready to show Dr. Pignier his changes. He brought a writing board carved with thin, horizontal grooves to their meeting in the director's office. He sat down opposite Dr. Pignier and placed a piece of paper on the board. Then he laid a sliding bar with tiny rectangular windows, each the size of a single cell, over the paper. Holding a pointed stylus in his hand, he asked Dr. Pignier to choose a book and to read a passage from it out loud.

The director chose a poem by Charles d'Orleans.

Time has lost her wintry gear
Of wind, and cold, and rain,
And is attired again
In radiant sunlight, bright and clear...

Braille punched the words quickly into his paper, and told the director that he could read faster.

When Dr. Pignier was finished, Braille turned the paper over and ran his fingers over the raised dots. He then steadily read every word the director had spoken, without one mistake.

Dr. Pignier was overcome with surprise and admiration. He rushed to Braille and embraced him. He promised to introduce the whole school to Braille's method.

At the time, Louis Braille was only fifteen years old.

Aa Bb Cc Dd Ee Ff Gg Hh Ii Jj

Kk Ll Mm Nn Oo Pp Qq Rr Ss Tt

Uu Vv Ww Xx Yy Zz

The Braille alphabet.

Courtesy of Perkins.

It would be wonderful to end Braille's story here. It would be nice to say that his dot system quickly spread throughout France and then the world.

But that is not how it happened.

The truth is that Braille fought his entire life to convince others that his system was a meaningful contribution to the blind. Many times he despaired that his system, though obviously superior to any other method, would ever be used by anyone outside the walls of his school, and sometimes, by anyone but himself. When Braille died in 1852, at the age of 43, he was practically unknown.

How did this happen? Braille's system was so simple to use. Blind people today cannot imagine life without it. Why did it take so long for braille to be fully adopted by others?

Braille's first setback occurred almost immediately. Dr. Pignier asked Captain Barbier to return to the school so that Braille could show him the modifications he'd made to make nightwriting more practical for blind people. Braille could barely contain his pride and excitement as he waited for the day to arrive. But when Braille showed the captain how he'd reduced the number of dots, eliminated the dashes, and made each cell represent a letter, rather than a sound, Barbier disapproved. He was insulted that a mere teenager would propose to change his system at all. He refused to consider any of Braille's ideas and angrily left the school.

Braille was devastated. No one had studied the dot system better than the captain and himself, and the older man's rejection was a terrible blow. But he wouldn't give up. In his diary he wrote, "If my eyes will not tell me about men and events, ideas and doctrines, I must find another way...If I cannot discover a way to read and write, to understand life about me and life from the past, then I shall kill myself."

Dr. Pignier, who did recognize the brilliant simplicity of Braille's method, decided to petition France's Interior Minister to consider adopting the dot system as the nation's official method of reading and writing for the blind. Although the Minister praised Braille's work, the government refused to discard the decades-old, official embossing system. How could a system devised by a mere boy be better than the established method, a system that, after all, was based on the letters of sighted people and allowed sighted people to better help the blind? Despite this setback, Dr. Pignier told Braille to remain hopeful. The French government had changed again and again for decades in the recurring struggle between Republicans and Royalists. Perhaps if they waited a few years, a new government, more receptive to the dot method, might come to power.

It was some solace to know that Braille's system was heartily adopted by his classmates. The boys began to keep diaries and write letters. Braille worked diligently to transcribe as many books as possible into the dot system. During this time he also became a talented musician and gained a degree of fame for being the resident organist at St. Nicholas Des-Champs, one of the most famous churches in Paris. He even devised a way to use the dots to write musical notes and notations.

In 1826, Dr. Pignier made seventeen-year-old Braille the first blind teacher at the Institute. Prior to this, the teachers had all been sighted, and it is important to note that many of them opposed Braille's dot system, which they had trouble learning. These teachers saw the dots as a "secret code" the students would use only amongst themselves. They believed Braille's system could make blind people give up trying to integrate with the outside world, and that if blind children gained too much knowledge from reading, they might be less content with their station in life. They feared the blind might begin to dream of doing more than knitting and sewing – of greater things, things the students would never be capable of achieving. What if more blind people became teachers? What if *all* the teachers were blind? The result would be a disaster, they thought. It would be the blind leading the blind – unthinkable.

Braille felt lucky to be a teacher at the school. The students loved him, for he could relate to them as none of the sighted teachers could, and it was common knowledge that he gave much of his earnings to cover poor students' tuition, never expecting to be repaid. When he wasn't teaching or playing music, he transcribed textbooks into dots for the students. He developed amazing reading speed approaching 2,500 dots per minute.

In 1829, Braille published a book entitled, *Method of Writing Words, Music and Plain Songs by Means of Dots, for use by the Blind and Arranged for Them*. In the preface, he gave credit to Captain Barbier by saying, "his method gave us the first idea of our own." Braille hoped this work would help promote the dot system outside of the school. He showed his technique to visitors with missionary zeal. He even demonstrated it to King Louis Philippe, among others, at the 1834 Exhibition of Industry held in the Place de la Concorde. The King complimented Braille, but nothing more came of the encounter.

While Braille was looking outward, searching for opportunities to spread his method to the world, he did not realize that the greatest challenge to the dot system would next come from within the school. Dr. Pignier had always been Braille's strongest advocate. In 1840, however, the old director was ousted by the maneuvering of his ambitious assistant, P. Armand Dufau. When he knew the political winds were in his favor, Dufau complained to the Minister of the Interior that Dr. Pignier was too liberal in his views toward education and further accused him of liberal political views that were sure to find disfavor in the current government. Whether or not Dr. Pignier actually held liberal views was immaterial. The accusation alone was enough to warrant dismissal by the Minister, and Monsieur Dufau became Director Dufau.

Dufau had always opposed Braille's system. He did not believe blind people should use an alphabet different from the one sighted people used. He sympathized with sighted teachers who worried they might lose their jobs if more blind students like Braille became teachers, or if the blind adopted a system of reading that the sighted teachers did not understand. Moreover, Dufau himself had invented a handguide that was designed to assist in the writing of embossed letters. This device would be useless if the dot system continued to spread.

The mood at the school changed overnight. Teachers began to enforce stricter discipline. The humor and mirth the students had enjoyed under Dr. Pignier disappeared. Then, Dufau banned the dot system entirely from the school. He seized all the books that had been transcribed into dots and confiscated the students' grooved slates and styluses. Most students continued to use the system in secret, using knitting needles, nails, forks, pencils, and anything else they could find to punch holes in paper. Older students taught the system to new, younger students. Whenever boys were caught using the dots, the teachers punished them by withholding meals or putting them into solitary confinement.

Braille grew despondent. As a teacher, he could not openly oppose the new director's mandate, and he worried that the dot method would be completely lost after he died. This concern was not too far-fetched, because Braille's health began to fail. For years he had been beset with a chronic, incessant cough. The cough appeared each year while he was at the school, and would improve each summer while at home in Coupvray getting fresh air and exercise in the countryside. In time he was diagnosed with consumption, later known as tuberculosis. This bacterial disease flourished in the damp and unsanitary conditions at the dilapidated Institute. Braille's health became so poor that, in 1843, he returned home for an extended stay of many months. Fortunately, after a long recuperation under the tender care of his mother, he improved.

But when Braille returned to Paris he learned that Director Dufau had done the unthinkable; in Braille's absence, he had ordered all the books that had been transcribed into the dot system be burned. Years of work, most of it done by Braille, were destroyed in a smoking bonfire in the school's courtyard. Braille was heartbroken.

It seemed that God had conspired to prevent Braille's system from ever reaching the outside world. Back at the school, he began to grow sick again. He feared that his life's work would count for nothing.

Finally, one man's decision changed the course of history for Braille and the blind. Director Dufau's assistant was a young man named Joseph Guadet. For years, Guadet had stood on the sidelines of the war between the teachers and students over the use of dots. Despite the crackdowns and punishments, the students continued to use the dot system, and in time, Guadet saw the brilliant simplicity of the method. He became the first sighted person to learn to read and write using Braille's method, and he realized the students would never let it be extinguished.

Guadet decided to tell this to Director Dufau. This was no small matter. He could lose his job for insubordination; the director was not known for being a forgiving man. Guadet carefully planned his approach. He explained to Director Dufau that the dots were by far the most efficient method of reading and writing ever devised for the blind. It would ultimately triumph, for there was no stopping it. Instead of opposing it, Dufau should embrace it, and gain credit for promoting it. Here was a chance for the director to become famous as the man who disseminated the dot system to the world. If Dufau did not claim credit now, someone else later would, and their school would be ridiculed for holding back the genius of one of its own students.

After a few days of careful consideration, Dufau came around to Guadet's reasoning. He reversed his decision to ban the dots. The students rejoiced.

In 1844, the Institute was moved to a brand new building, a grand and spacious edifice that can still be seen today. At the opening ceremony, on February 22, 1844, Director Dufau let Guadet surprise the assembled crowd by announcing that there would be a public demonstration of a new system of writing for the blind, based on dots. Guadet chose a volunteer from the audience and invited the man to the stage. He asked the volunteer to read aloud from a book of poetry while a young blind girl transcribed his words into dots. When the recitation was finished, a second blind girl who had been kept out of earshot in another room entered, took the paper from the first girl, and read the poem aloud perfectly, word for word.

A resounding swell of applause erupted from the audience. However, one government official in the crowd challenged the demonstration. He questioned whether the girl had simply memorized the poem.

Guadet invited the official to read from anything he chose.

The man reached into his pocket and withdrew a ticket stub. From it, he read the name of a musical performance he had attended, its date, time, and location. This time, the second blind girl transcribed the words while the first one was kept outside the room. When the first girl entered and repeated the words perfectly, the audience roared its approval.

Guadet invited Braille to stand and be acknowledged as the inventor of the system. *Braille,* as the dot system came to be called, would thereafter be adopted by the Institute.

Louis Braille succumbed to tuberculosis on January 6, 1852. He died with no fanfare and not one newspaper article in France marked his passing. His body was taken to Coupvray to be buried near his family home. He never lived to see braille spread beyond the walls of his school.

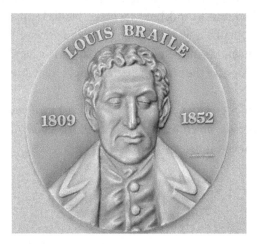

Louis Braille commemorative medal, sculpted by Humberto Mendes.

Courtesy of the Museum of Vision and the American Academy of Ophthalmology. All rights reserved.

Two years after Braille's death, braille was officially adopted by the French government. Over the next twenty-five years, other European nations recognized and adopted it as well. The United States was one of the last western nations to do so, in 1917. In 1949, the United Nations proposed a standardized version that could be used around the world.

Braille has now permitted millions of visually-impaired people to read and write. It has been adapted to Chinese characters and African ideograms. Computers can quickly transcribe and print books in braille. There are braille keyboards and braille libraries.

Louis Braille's dream has come true.

In 1952, Louis Braille's body was carefully exhumed from the village of Coupvray and transported for reburial at the Pantheon in Paris. At the commemoration ceremony, Helen Keller said, "... we, the blind, are as indebted to Louis Braille as mankind is to Gutenberg." Braille now rests among France's greatest heroes, such as Curie, Hugo, Voltaire, Rousseau, and Zola. His hands, however, the hands that gave the blind their greatest gift, remain enshrined in Coupvray.

His family's grey stone house is now a museum. If you visit it, you will see a plaque which reads, "He opened the doors of knowledge to all those who cannot see."

Chapter Nine

VISIONARIES

"**A**re you *sure* you haven't been hit in the eye?" I asked Ann, the quiet eighteen-year-old sitting in my exam chair. She was Asian-American, slightly overweight, and obviously very shy.

Ann pursed her lips and stared at her shoes for a moment. Her father sat behind me, against the wall and below the screen where the eye chart was projected. He leaned forward and said quietly, "Well, were you?"

Ann shook her head slowly from side to side. She seemed to consider this question very hard, even though she'd already answered negatively the first time around.

"And you don't have diabetes or any blood clotting disorders?" I asked.

"No, she doesn't," Dad said.

I nodded and looked at Ann's left eye again through the slit lamp. The anterior chamber was filled with blood, a *total hyphema*. An ultrasound of the eye had revealed a dense vitreous hemorrhage and severe retinal detachment.

"And you said it's been blurry like this for at least three weeks already?" The most she could see with this eye was my hand waving in front of her face.

"Yes," Ann said.

I sat back and swung the slit lamp out of the way.

"I asked about trauma, Ann, because it's quite unusual for a young person like you to get a spontaneous retinal detachment as severe as this, and with so much bleeding." I paused for a moment, again leaving an opening for Ann to respond, but she remained silent.

"Whatever the cause, you're in a difficult spot. I can do surgery to wash out the blood and fix your detachment, but right now the blood is blocking my view of the retina so it's hard for me to see the extent of the damage. I can't tell you how much vision you might expect to get back."

I went over more details about the operation and recovery with Ann and her father. They consented to the surgery and signed the paperwork.

Neither Ann, nor I, knew that this would only be the beginning of her troubles.

The blood inside her eye was thick, with many clots – the way blood looks after it's been congealing for a while. I carefully evacuated the maroon, glutinous blobs. The blood was so thickly plastered against the back of her lens that it was going to be impossible to clear it off without touching the lens and giving her a cataract, so I decided to remove the lens with an ultrasonic probe.

After clearing more blood, I got a view of the detachment.

Wow.

It was impressive. The retina was totally detached. Instead of just one discrete retinal tear, the retina had actually become circumferentially *dis-inserted* from its root just behind the iris, near the front of the eye. For three clock hours, from 9 o'clock to 12 o'clock, the torn edge of Ann's retina was beginning to curl up on itself like a scroll, a *retinal dialysis*.

This type of detachment is often seen after significant trauma.

But she'd said there wasn't any trauma. I'd asked her twice.

And now I saw a new problem.

A much bigger problem.

The retina at the bottom of Ann's eye was blanketed by sheets of fibrotic scar tissue, which were pulling on the retina and lifting it so that the whole complex looked like a taut trampoline.

I groaned.

We have a name for this type of tissue reaction: *proliferative vitreoretinopathy*, usually seen in chronic, severe detachments. It's the most common cause of postoperative re-detachment – a.k.a. surgical failure.

Imagine you're a contestant on the game show *Minute to Win It*, the one in which you win money by performing silly tasks like stacking seven ding-dongs on your forehead, or balancing six dice on a popsicle stick held in your mouth, or bouncing quarters off a table and into the top of a water jug positioned several feet away. Now, imagine you are presented with a single layer of scrunched-up tissue paper, and it stays scrunched up because someone has stuck several pieces of scotch tape across the top of it. Using one pair of tweezers, your task is to gently peel off the pieces of scotch tape so that you can smooth out and flatten the tissue paper. You lose if: the tissue paper gets torn, you can't peel off all the scotch tape, or you run out of time.

This is like what I'd need to do to flatten Ann's retina. And remember, the retina is delicate neural tissue packed with sight-giving photoreceptors. It's only 250 microns thick, just one-fourth of one millimeter. *Any* manipulation of it is certain to cause some damage.

I was going to have to dissect off loads of "scotch tape" while causing as little harm as possible.

I spent a lot of time trying to do just this. The entire effort was racked with tension – like the ophthalmological equivalent of scraping tumor cells off of the parts of the brain that control speech or memory. I was walking through a minefield: a tentative tug on a membrane with my microforceps, a decision to pull a little harder to try and get it off, a sigh of relief to see the retina hadn't been ripped, then the disheartening prospect of needing to do it again, and again. Then, it inevitably happened: as I gently peeled one membrane and lifted it up to see how adherent it was, the retina tore. The tear was jagged, like a rip in one of my old T-shirts.

My shoulders slumped.

So much for perfection.

I tried to focus. This was taking a long time, well over an hour already, and I was going to have to get moving. I tried to work faster, continuing to peel, tease, and coax the membranes off the retina. At some point, I discovered there were also membranes affixed to the *underside* of Ann's retina. To remove those, I had to make *intentional* holes in the retina and pass my forceps through the holes to try and peel them off from behind. The bottom half of the retina was starting to look like Swiss cheese. It was laborious and unsatisfying work.

Once I'd finally peeled off as many membranes as possible, it was time to see if I'd done enough. I injected perfluoron® into the eye, a liquid heavy enough to flatten the retina beneath it. If I'd removed enough scar tissue, and made the retina free enough, it ought to flatten completely.

I injected the heavy liquid slowly. The macula went flat, and – *wait* – I looked closer. *What is that? A hole?*

It was a macular hole.

How the hell did she get a macular hole?

Macular holes occur in older people, or – I knew – after trauma. Now I *knew* Ann had probably gotten hit in this eye, somehow, somewhere. I grew concerned – *had someone been hurting her?* She had seemed to be on guard…but about what?

I took a deep breath and pushed this thought from my mind. There was no time to dwell on it now. I was in salvage mode. I knew I'd be lucky just to get her retina flat.

When I finished injecting the perfluoron bubble, I realized it wasn't going to work.

The bottom half of her retina still wasn't flat. It remained too scarred, too rigid, and too taut to flatten. Everything I'd done up to this point had gotten me no closer to my goal. And worse, Ann's cornea was getting hazy, which can happen during a lengthy surgery. My view through it was becoming foggy. I was running out of time.

There was one option left. I had to cut the retina.

Imagine you're told to cut a globe in half, so that you are only holding the western hemisphere. Then you place this on a table, so it's sitting there like a bowl, and you're told to completely flatten the earth's surface onto the table. You see at once that this is impossible because the globe is too rigid and won't fully flatten no matter how much you press on one area. The only way to do it is to cut the globe, to make *relaxing* incisions. This will damage it, of course. Antarctica and northern Canada are going to come out looking pretty distorted, but they'll have to be sacrificed to achieve the greater good.

To get the retina at the bottom of Ann's eye to flatten, I was going to have to cut it, destroying the very tissue I'd spent so long trying to carefully protect.

I cauterized a swath of retina where I intended to cut so it wouldn't bleed. Then I started cutting with my vitrector, eating up 180 degrees of peripheral retina in a large semi-circle, like the mouth of a smiley face. In contrast to the delicate surgery I'd done up to that point, this act was purely destructive. But now the retina did lay flat, though it was severely foreshortened. I applied laser treatment generously to the cut edge of retina, praying the laser scars would be strong enough to affix the retina to the eye wall after it healed.

At the end of the surgery I filled Ann's eye with an oil bubble, which would help hold the retina in place until I removed the oil in another surgery months later.

I was done. I'd spent over two hours – a long time for an eye surgery – working to get Ann's retina to look halfway decent. It was flat, at least for now.

Ann's retina was flat the next day, and at the following visit, a week later. I'd instructed her to remain face-down the entire week, no easy task. This position made the bubble, which floats skyward, exert the most pressure on both the bottom half of the retina and the macular hole.

During these visits, Ann seemed withdrawn. I privately asked her if anyone had hurt her. She said no. I took her father aside and asked him if there was any possibility that someone might be harming her, but he said this was impossible – she spent almost all her time alone in her bedroom. I called her primary care doctor to let him know what I'd found. He said he'd bring her in for an evaluation to investigate it further and, if necessary, set up a meeting with a social worker.

Meantime, the retina stayed flat past the one month point, then two months, then three. Her macular hole closed. Everything was looking good. I was beginning to believe we'd fixed her retina, and we began to prepare for the next step, to remove her oil bubble. After that, she could get an artificial lens, and then, who knew what her vision might be?

One day, about four months after her left eye surgery, Ann and her father returned to my office for an unscheduled visit. I noticed her dad was leading her by the arm as they came down the hallway.

"My right eye's blurry now," she told me as she felt her way into the exam chair.

What?

The right eye had always seen 20/20. Today it was 20/400.

I looked inside.

Oh no.

The right retina was totally detached. There were four clock-hours of retinal dialysis laterally.

Something is very wrong here, I thought.

"Ann," I said gravely. "You've got another terrible detachment. Now you're legally blind in both eyes. I can't believe this just happened spontaneously – you still say you haven't had any trauma?"

Ann looked at her shoes, didn't say a word.

Her father cleared his throat. "Well…we've got something new to tell you, Dr. Lam. It's something that's been difficult for all of us… at home." He was speaking slowly, pausing, and suddenly I noticed how tired he looked. "Ann's been seeing a psychiatrist," he said.

"Why?" I asked tentatively.

"We've, um, found her doing something at night."

"Like what?"

"We think she's doing it in her sleep. We think she's…"

He paused. I held my breath.

"Poking her eyes."

"Poking…her…eyes?"

"Yes, very hard. We saw her doing it." He demonstrated by rapidly jabbing his thumbs at his eyes. "The psychiatrist thinks she doesn't remember it after it happens. Could this explain what's been happening to her eyes?"

Oh my God.

"Yes, it probably does."

I can't believe she's doing this to herself. This nice kid. Now both eyes ruined.

It was a tragedy.

We sat in silence for a while, and the gravity of what he'd told me slowly sunk in. Poor Ann. We talked for a while about her condition. I was glad she didn't have any other physical injuries. They were moving her bed into her parents' room. The psychiatrist was going to monitor her closely.

I brought the discussion back to her eye. "Our backs are against the wall, Ann. This detachment in your right eye is pretty bad, almost as bad as your left eye was. I can't promise how well this will turn out, but I think we've got to try to fix it."

"Okay," Ann said timidly.

The operation on her right eye went smoothly. The retina showed some early signs of proliferative vitreoretinopathy and scar tissue, but nothing nearly as severe as what had afflicted her left eye. I filled the eye with an oil bubble and told her to lie on her left side for a week.

I watched her closely for the next several weeks. The right retina stayed flat. During this time she could barely see out of either eye, and therefore was completely dependent on her family to help her accomplish daily tasks or leave their home.

One day, about a month after the right eye's surgery, I re-examined her left eye, the first eye I'd operated on, and noticed something was different.

The left retina was re-detaching.

It wasn't a dramatic change. There was still an oil bubble in the eye keeping the retina mostly flat, but at the bottom of the eye, the cut edge of retina was lifting up, new scar tissue was forming, and fluid was getting under the macula.

"Your retina is re-detaching in the left eye," I told her. "We can do another surgery to remove the oil, flatten the retina again, and put oil back in."

"Would I have to be face-down again?"

"Yes, for a week."

"Will it work?"

"I don't know. I hope so, but I can't guarantee it."

She and her father agreed to try.

In this surgery I had to cut away more of the scarred retina to flatten it. I re-filled the eye with oil. I sent her home and told her to do her best to position face-down.

For a while, it looked pretty good. We had agreed to leave the oil bubble in for at least six months, and everything was fine after two months, and then three months. But after four months, it was clear the retina was detaching yet again. Same problem: scar tissue – thick, fibrous, and adherent to what was left of the retina below the macula.

I was crestfallen. We were back to square one, all the worse because of everything Ann had already endured. I stood over Ann for a few moments in the dark exam room, keeping the news of her re-detachment to myself for the moment because I knew it would devastate both of them. They were hoping for another good report. I dreaded delivering the bad news.

And what should I tell them? Should I try to fix it again? It would be her fourth surgery. At this point, there wasn't much retina left to work with. The scarring was up into the macula and I couldn't cut or laser the macula. In fact, even if I *could* flatten her retina, I wasn't sure if her vision would be significantly better than it was right now – just counting fingers. Should I expose her again to all the risks of surgery? They weren't insignificant: bleeding, infection, pain, high eye pressure, and rarely, complete blindness or loss of the eye.

I told them what had happened. We talked for a long time, and I explained the risks and benefits of another surgery. I told them I wasn't sure if we should operate and I asked them what they wanted to do.

"I don't know," Ann said.

Her dad was almost at a loss for words.

"Please tell us what to do," he said.

What if this were my eye? I asked myself. I guessed the chances of fixing it were less than thirty percent. And even if I succeeded, I thought it was unlikely that she would ever be able to see more than the big "E" on the chart with this eye.

But...there was always a chance...

The retina fellowship where I trained is widely considered to be among the best in the country. A surgeon-in-training at a good vitreo-retinal surgical fellowship might perform or participate in 400-500 surgeries over the course of two years. I did about 1,200. But, having confidence in my ability to perform any surgical maneuver did not make me a great surgeon. There was still something important I lacked: the years of experience that might help me make the best possible decision for Ann.

It has been said that the difference between a good surgeon and a great surgeon is that a great surgeon knows when *not* to operate. That day, sitting with Ann and her dad as they anxiously waited for me to decide whether we should re-operate, I fully appreciated the wisdom of this statement. Oftentimes in medicine, the right choice is obvious. If you've got a broken arm, you undergo surgery to fix it. If you're in labor and your baby's heart rate is dropping, you consent to a C-section to get the baby out. But at other times, a decision can be far more difficult. Ann's case was one of those times – when it wasn't clear if the benefit of surgery outweighed the risk.

It's funny, because I used to think it would be nice to have patients who'd say to me, "You're the expert, Doc. I trust you. Just tell me what to do." But now I know that that's when the surgeon feels the weight of responsibility most heavily.

It's far easier when, after discussing the pros and cons of a surgery, patients tell me what they want to do.

But sometimes, they can't make a decision.

And sometimes, there is no right or wrong choice.

———

I'd had doubts up until the last moment. We were in the pre-op area and Ann was obviously trying to be brave, while her dad tried not to show how worried he was. I thought about how difficult I knew her surgery was going to be, and about having her position face-down again for another week, and about all the post-operative visits and possible problems that might make me regret re-operating on this eye.

I almost asked them again, "Are you *sure* you want to do this?"

But then I remembered, they weren't sure, they'd told me as much. They'd asked *me* what to do.

There wasn't anything scientific about my decision to try again. No article in any medical journal could tell me what the right decision was. For me, it came down to one thought. *If we do the surgery, we'll know we tried and did everything we could.* I'd asked myself what I would do in her position and I decided that I wouldn't want to spend the next sixty years wondering, *what if I'd tried, would it have been possible to see any better with this eye?*

The conjunctiva was scarred from her previous surgeries. I carefully examined her sclera to identify the old incision sites so I could avoid them with the new ones. I inserted a cannula and extracted the oil from her eye. Then I inserted my light pipe and took a look.

I knew almost immediately that Ann's chances for improved vision were even worse than I'd thought. Now, in the absence of the oil bubble which had kept much of the retina flat and looking somewhat decent, I could see that the retina was not only everywhere detached but also *atrophic* and probably *ischemic* – thinned and dead from lack of blood flow. Still, I started to work, thinking that a flat almost-dead retina might be better than a detached almost-dead retina. Just below the macula, the scarred tissue was so thick that this time I couldn't even cut its edge with my vitrector. I twanged the edge of the detachment, its consistency reminiscent of cardboard. I tried intraocular scissors, and even these were not strong enough to break the thickest cords of disfigured tissue. After a few more minutes of probing, peeling, and attempts at cutting, I stopped.

I just stared at the retina, I'm not sure for how long. Some areas were barely recognizable as retina at all – distorted by traction or charred from previous laser treatment. To flatten it this time, I'd have to sacrifice part of the macula, the inviolate, precious macula. And even if I did that, I doubted I could succeed. I could spend hours peeling, dissecting, praying – but to what end? Would it do Ann any good? Would she see any better?

"Dr. Lam?"

Someone was speaking to me. I blinked, turned my head.

"Dr. Lam? What are you doing?"

It was my assistant. She was staring at me. So was the circulating nurse and the anesthesiologist.

I turned back to the scope. "I'm *thinking*," I said.

I had to decide whether to keep working or throw in the towel.

For a while the only sound was the dutiful beeping of the anesthesiologist's machines.

I decided to close up.

It was un-fixable.

This was the first time I'd been unable to fix a retinal detachment. Up to that point, I'd always succeeded, though it may have taken three, or even four surgeries, I'd always gotten the retina flat. I'm sure it was inevitable that I'd eventually encounter a case like Ann's, but this didn't make my disappointment any easier to bear.

Afterwards, I had a long talk with Ann and her dad, explaining what I'd seen, and why I wasn't going to be able to fix her left eye.

They understood.

They were grateful we had tried again.

———

Medicine will never be perfect. There will always be diseases that evade our best treatments and afflictions that exceed our ability to fix or to heal. We live along a continuum of medical progress. When viewed over the course of human history, the pace of this progress has dramatically spiked in the last fifty years with the explosion of new discoveries and advanced treatments that we enjoy today. Will the future of medicine continue ascending on this trajectory?

It would be a mistake to assume that it will. When Americans watched Neil Armstrong and Buzz Aldrin walk on the moon in 1969, they marveled. Less than ten years had elapsed from Alan Shepard's first foray into space to landing on the moon. If you asked an American in 1969 what he or she thought we might achieve in space exploration over the next forty years, most of them probably would have assumed we'd have gotten to Mars and maybe beyond. Those forty years have passed. Progress doesn't always proceed at the pace we expect or hope for.

Future medical discoveries will depend on the work of individual doctors and scientists, just as it always has. It won't happen just because the government increases funding for science, or because of pharmaceutical companies that throw their weight behind the search for the next wonder drug. The breakthroughs will come from physicians and researchers who share the qualities of the heroes in these pages: determination, perseverance, a dissatisfaction with the status quo, and a willingness to take risks. Surely these are the traits that parents and teachers should seek to nurture in today's students – the young people we'll rely upon for tomorrow's discoveries. They will be the ones who may someday be able to offer patients like Ann a different, better outcome than we can provide today.

In hindsight, visionaries like Harold Ridley, Charles Kelman, Judah Folkman, and the rest may seem larger than life. Their discoveries improved the sight of millions around the world, and time has a way of imparting mythical qualities to the work of our heroes. But we should not forget that these were ordinary men, born into humble circumstances, who made mistakes, faced opposition, and failed repeatedly. They were not so different from the rest of us in many respects, for though they made extraordinary discoveries, we're all capable of emulating the qualities that led to their achievements. They shared a passion for saving sight, and their lives remind us that our own passions, whatever they are, can enable us to offer our own improvements to the world.

It's obvious, in retrospect, that Ann's last operation did not help her. I asked myself, if I'd had more experience, if I'd previously operated on many other difficult cases like Ann's, could I have known ahead of time that it would be futile to try to fix her again?

I don't know the answer to this, even now. I'm sure additional experience could have helped me make the decision, just as I'm sure Ann's case will inform my recommendations to similar patients in the future. But the more I turned it over and over in my mind, the more I knew that I'd make the same choice again. And twenty years from now, when another eighteen-year-old Ann is sitting across from me and I know the odds of success are very long indeed, if there's still a chance of improvement, and the patient wants to, I know I'll try.

Thankfully, the detachment in her right eye fared much better. This retina remained flat after I removed the oil bubble. She later had cataract surgery and her vision improved to 20/25.

Now she's able to see well enough to succeed in school and work at almost any job. She's closely followed by her psychiatrist and hasn't had any recurrence of self-harmful behavior.

There is nothing more I can do for Ann's worse, left eye today, but she's still a young woman, and no doubt in our lifetimes, we will see more amazing advances in my field. In fact, it's quite probable that the treatments I'll be doing in twenty years will hardly resemble the ones I do today. Already, blind patients with a condition called *retinitis pigmentosa* are receiving implants of sight-giving retinal microchips, a treatment the FDA approved in February 2013. These patients wear special glasses fitted with a miniature camera. The image captured by the camera is converted into a series of electrical pulses which are transmitted wirelessly to a microchip that is surgically affixed to the macula; the chip then stimulates the retina's remaining cells to send visual signals to the brain. At present, the chip is only a 60-electrode array; but already, previously blind or near-blind patients have been able to distinguish light and dark, detect movement, navigate around large obstacles, and read largely printed words.

In the future, we'll probably employ gene therapy to stop or prevent diseases like macular degeneration. Instead of monthly injections of Avastin® or Lucentis®, we might inject tiny, inactivated viruses to transport specially-engineered genes which promote the production of proteins that inhibit photoreceptor degradation, or block the proliferation of harmful cell products. Someday we might be able to prevent wet macular degeneration altogether. Clinicians have already begun a human clinical trial using gene therapy to treat a rare blinding condition called *Leber's congenital amaurosis*, after a similar treatment successfully restored some sight to blind dogs afflicted with the same genetic defect.

The use of stem cells holds promise as well. Human embryonic stem cells have the ability to develop into any cell-type in the body, and already, researchers have demonstrated success at coaxing stem cells to perform the same functions as cells that make up the retinal pigment epithelium, an important layer of the retina. The FDA recently approved the first human clinical trial using these cells. Someday, stem cells might be used to treat virtually any degenerative retinal disease.

And these are only the treatments we can imagine today. To be sure, there will be other miraculous therapies which we cannot even begin to fathom now – just as Harold Ridley would never have dreamed something like LASIK surgery could exist. The men and women who discover such treatments will, no doubt, be dedicated visionaries. Their new ideas may prompt their peers to label them heretics, or they might be recognized as heroes. We do not know how they will affect our collective futures, but we can be sure that whoever they are, they will succeed because of an inner drive, a passion, that makes giving up impossible. And most likely, their passion will be no different than that of their predecessors: to help people.

Sometimes, young people ask me for advice about going to, or getting into, medical school. This commonly comes up during the college admissions interviews I conduct locally for my undergraduate alma mater. The first thing I make sure to tell these high schoolers is to ask themselves if they want to help people.

"Forget about what you think others want to hear," I'll tell them, "or what you think sounds good in an interview. Ask yourself, 'Do I truly enjoy helping people?'"

Because unless the answer is an unequivocal "yes," he or she may regret a decision to become a physician. The journey can take over a decade of arduous training. The hours are long and stressful.

And, there are other, easier ways of making money. I know some doctors, friends of mine, who wouldn't choose medicine if given the chance to start again. Some of them became doctors because they wanted to please their parents. Others went to medical school because, at the time, they couldn't think of anything they might like better. All of these friends are excellent doctors – smart, competent, and empathetic. Yet, now that they're practicing, they aren't entirely happy because their true passion lay elsewhere. Plenty of them still wanted to help people, but would have preferred to do it as a pastor, a public servant, or a businessperson. Some of them realized that their life's greatest fulfillment would come from raising children and not from working full-time in a demanding profession. Others regretted not working harder to find or develop their true passion for writing, music, or art.

I'm sure my advice seems abstract to the nervous applicants I meet, most of whom are trying very hard to make a good impression. To be sure, many of them probably don't know what they're passionate about, but I make sure to tell them that's normal. It can take a very long time, sometimes most of a lifetime, to find out what's most important to each of us.

"Just remember," I tell them, "stay curious, don't be satisfied with the way things are, dream of how you can make things better. Even if you've started down one path, it's never too late to change course if you discover your passion."

I think of the visionaries in this book, and I make sure to add, "And if you find it, do it. It'll make you happy, and you might just accomplish something great."

ACKNOWLEDGMENTS

I must first thank my patients, many of whom inspire me by their serenity and courage in the face of sometimes difficult circumstances. I am continually humbled by the trust and confidence they so readily confer upon physicians like myself. Being a part of their lives is truly a privilege.

Gerald Hausman, my friend and editor, deserves the credit for convincing me to write this book. I'd just finished writing my first novel when he told me, "You should really write that eye book next." But the history of ophthalmology did not strike me as something most people would be interested in. "So make it *interesting,*" he said. I thank him for his persistence and for the multitude of other things he's done to help bring this book to life.

I also owe thanks to Stephany Evans, literary agent, who believed in this book, took it on, and helped me view it with a more critical eye. Her enthusiasm gave me confidence that it would find a ready audience.

Every surgeon is the product of his or her teachers. I am indebted to scores of physicians and surgeons who taught and trained me, or worked beside me as colleagues. Several generously gave of their time to help improve this manuscript, including: William Tasman, Julia Haller, Joan Miller, Peter Laibson, Chris Rapuano, David Pao, Bradley Foster, and David Agahigian.

For their valuable support and assistance, deep thanks also go to Nicholas Ridley, Ann Kelman, Paula Folkman, Ellen Patz, Rafe Sagalyn, Chris Min Park, Alice Tasman, Richard Wilbur, Robert Bagg, Lorry Hausman, Jenny Benjamin, Debra Marchi, Todd Lajoie, the staff of Baystate Medical Center's Health Sciences Library, and especially to Katherine Lu and Mariah Fox.

I am grateful to my father, Wilfred Lam, whose example showed me how fulfilling a life in medicine could be; to my mother, Esther Lam, whose love of history inspired my own; and finally, to my wife, Christina, for enduring years of medical training by my side, for suffering through early drafts, and for everything else that really matters.

NOTES

Chapter Two | *"This operation should never be done."*
Harold Ridley and the Intraocular Lens

21   *the invention of one man, Harold Ridley:* The author thanks Mr. Nicholas
      Ridley, Sir Ridley's son, for reviewing this chapter and for offering
      valuable insight into his father's career and personal life. The author
      also acknowledges the late Dr. David Apple, Harold Ridley's personal
      friend and official biographer, for his years of work spent researching
      Sir Ridley's life, and for his longstanding efforts to bring attention to
      Sir Ridley's remarkable accomplishments.

22   *RAF Airbase at Tangmere:* This account of Gordon "Mouse" Cleaver's
      dogfight on August 15, 1940, is primarily based on an historical
      account of the battle in Dr. David Apple's biography of Harold Ridley
      (Apple, David J. *Sir Harold Ridley and His Fight for Sight.* Thorofare,
      NJ; Slack, 2006: 111-120.). While Dr. Apple based his account
      on interviews with a member of Cleaver's family and pilots of his
      squadron, Flight Lieutenant Cleaver never published his own, first-
      hand account of combat, and hence, it must be acknowledged that

the thoughts, dialogue, and some details of what is presented here are fictional. We *do* know that Cleaver landed after a mid-day sortie and had just sat down to mess hall refreshments when the pilots were called to scramble quickly again. His plane was not ready, so he took off in a new Hurricane, and in his haste, forgot to bring his protective goggles. We also know that, when he was shot down, his canopy shattered and shards of plexiglass penetrated his eyes, and that he, now sightless, unbuckled his harness and rolled the plane to fall out of it. Cleaver was a member of the famed No. 601 "Millionaires' Squadron." He was ultimately credited with seven total kills and received the Distinguished Flying Cross. Before the war he had represented Britain in international skiing competitions. Max Aitken was a highly respected squadron leader of the No. 601 Squadron.

Michael Korda's book about the Battle of Britain (Korda, Michael. *With Wings Like Eagles: The Untold Story of the Battle of Britain.* New York, NY; Harper Perennial, 2009.) was helpful in providing a sense of what combat was like for Hurricane pilots in the summer of 1940.

28   *largest air battle in history:* Korda, Michael. *With Wings Like Eagles: The Untold Story of the Battle of Britain* (New York, NY; Harper Perennial, 2009), 177.

28   *involving over a thousand warplanes:* Ibid., 189.

28   *He would later undergo:* Apple, David J. *Sir Harold Ridley and His Fight for Sight* (Thorofare, NJ; Slack, 2006), 121.

28   *soft spoken, unassuming young ophthalmologist:* Nicholas Ridley. Personal communication, February 27, 2013.

29   *for someone like Ridley to challenge:* Apple DJ. Sir Nicolas Harold Ridley: 'All's Well That Ends Well.' Amer J Ophthalmol 2002; 133(1): 131-132.

30   *His father, Nicholas, had served:* Apple DJ, Sims J. Harold Ridley and the Invention of the Intraocular Lens. Surv Ophth 1996; 40(4): 280.

30   *the "lost generation":* Apple, *Sir Ridley,* 48.

31   *Amazingly, it [couching] is still performed:* Chan C. Couching for Cataract in China. Surv Ophthalmol 2010; 55(4); 393-398.

31   *He made an enemy:* Apple, *Sir Ridley,* 158.

32   *"Obviously something had to be done":* Apple DJ, Sims J 1996: 281.

32   *he also insisted that all consultants:* Nicholas Ridley. Personal commun-

ication, February 28, 2013.

32   *He felt the first impact:* Apple, *Sir Ridley,* 158.

33   *Ridley wrote, "This distressed me":* Ibid., 48-49.

33   *With time on his hands, Ridley dedicated:* Ridley, Harold. Ocular Onchocerciasis. Br J Ophthalmol 1945; Monograph Supplement.

33   *Ridley described the condition:* Ridley, Harold. Ocular manifestations of malnutrition in released prisoners of war from Thailand. Br J Ophthalmol 1945; December: 613-618.

33   *"I treated over 200 released allied prisoners of war":* Apple DJ, Sims J 1996: 282.

34   *he'd treated RAF pilots:* Apple, *Sir Ridley,* 109.

34   *"Jack, tell them all":* Ibid., 121.

34   *"unless a sharp edge of the plastic material":* Apple DJ, Sims J 1996: 285.

35   *"extraction alone is but half the cure for cataract":* Ridley, Harold. Intra-ocular acrylic lenses after cataract extraction. Lancet 1952; Jan 19; 1(6699): 118-121.

35   *"Mr. Ridley, it's a pity":* Apple DJ, Sims J 1996: 284.

35   *"While seated in the car":* Apple, *Sir Ridley,* 135.

36   *Ridley scheduled the first patient:* Choyce DP. Harold Ridley's First Patient. J Cataract Refract Surg 1999; 25: 731.

36   *"We must not fail to honor":* Apple, *Sir Ridley,* 141.

37   *One of Ridley's patients:* Ibid., 151.

37   *Critics excoriated him:* Ibid., 153.

37   *"In spite of my request":* Apple DJ, Sims J 1996: 287.

38   *"There was, however":* Rosen E, Phillipson B. Gullstrand lecture, Stockholm 1992: Mr. Harold Ridley. European Journal of Implant and Refractive Surgery 1993; 5: 4-7.

38   *"When the presentation of the paper ended":* Apple, *Sir Ridley,* 159.

38   *Comments from his peers included:* Moore DB, Harris A, Siesky B. The world through a lens: the vision of Sir Harold Ridley. Br J Ophthalmol 2010; 94: 1278.

39   *a close friend of Duke-Elder's:* Apple, *Sir Ridley,* 50.

39   *"In spite of Mr. Ridley's":* Vail D. Discussion of Ridley H: Further observations on intraocular acrylic lenses in cataract surgery. Trans Am Acad Ophthalmol Otolaryngol 1953; Jan-Feb: 99.

39   *Ridley once recalled:* Apple DJ, Sims J 1996: 288-289.

40   *"Many ophthalmologists and their patients":* Ibid., 289.

40   *"put out to pasture":* Apple, *Sir Ridley,* 162.

40   *"Let me tell you":* Ibid., 177.

40   *"I recall him as a slight man":* Walker C. Harold Ridley – Surgeon and Visionary. Southampton Medical Journal 1986; 3(1): 18.

41   *"Harold's method of teaching":* Ibid., 18-19.

41   *"delayed the cure of aphakia":* Apple, *Sir Ridley,* 11.

42   *It is estimated:* Taylor HR. Cataract: how much surgery do we have to do? Br J Ophthalmol; 84: 2.

43   *In 1987, the traumatic cataract:* Apple, *Sir Ridley,* 121.

Chapter Three | *"The delicious sensation of that ultrasonic probe against my teeth…"*
Charles Kelman and Phacoemulsification

49   *"Yes, one guy, but he was really interesting,":* The author is grateful to Mrs. Ann Kelman, Dr. Kelman's widow, for reviewing this chapter and for contributing useful insight into her husband's family life, medical career, and passion for music.

49   *New York City, 1965:* This account of Charles Kelman's epiphany at his dentist's office and struggle to invent phacoemulsifiation is drawn from his autobiography (Kelman, Charles D. *Through My Eyes: The story of a surgeon who dared to take on the medical world.* New York; Crown, 1985: 6, 9, 32-35, 61-69, 75-83, 92-98, 102-109.). However, it should be noted that portions of the narrative, including the description of the dentist's office and some of the subject's thoughts, are fictional.

50   *His father always dispensed advice:* Ann Kelman. Personal communication, February 27, 2013.

52   *His first experiments were on cats:* Kelman CD, Cooper IS. Cryosurgery of Retinal Detachment and other Ocular Conditions. Eye, ear, nose & throat monthly 1965; 42: 42-46.

56   *"I knew it wouldn't be quite that easy"*: Kelman, Charles D. *Through My Eyes: The story of a surgeon who dared to take on the medical world* (New York; Crown, 1985), 109.

57   *Kelman's next move:* Ibid., 109-112.

57   *This was about the fortieth prototype:* Oransky, Ivan. Charles Kelman. Lancet 2004; 364: 134.

57   *"At the end of two years"*: Kelman CD. The History and Development of Phacoemulsification. Int Ophthalmol Clin 1994; 34(2): 3.

58   *His first patient was John Martin:* Kelman, *Through My Eyes*, 122-129.

59   *"I looked at the eye"*: Ibid., 129.

59   *He pinpointed the problem:* Ibid., 130-133.

59   *Finally, he found a company:* Kelman CD. The genesis of phaco-emulsification. Cat Refract Surg Today 2004; March: 57-58.

60   *He found a new patient:* Kelman, *Through My Eyes*, 137-140.

60   *One day, Kelman operated on:* Ibid., 143-150.

63   *"Phaco is OK", "Phaco causes glaucoma", "Anyone over age 30"*: Kratz R. From von Graefe to Kelman. Cat Refract Surg Today 2004; March: 56.

63   *"Cataract surgery has been developed"*: Pandey SK, Milverton EJ, Maloof AK. A tribute to Charles David Kelman, MD: ophthalmologist, inventor and pioneer of phacoemulsification surgery. Clin & Exp Ophth 2004; 32: 531.

Chapter Four | *"I did not want to be considered a military hero."*
Charles Schepens and the Binocular Indirect Ophthalmoscope

73   *July 21, 1943:* This portrayal of the day Charles Schepens was confronted by the Gestapo is based on the account contained in Meg Ostrum's biography of Dr. Schepens (Ostrum, Meg. *The Surgeon and the Shepherd: Two Resistance Heroes in Vichy France*. Lincoln, NE; University of Nebraska Press, 2004: 114-127.). Although the narrative is based in fact, the author's dramatization is fictional. In addition, the author is indebted to Dr. William Tasman (former Chairman of Wills Eye Hospital), who trained under Dr. Schepens as a retina fellow, for sharing memories related to him by Dr. Schepens about the invention of the indirect ophthalmoscope and Dr. Schepens' post-war career.

79   *"At the time, I even had the idea"*: Oransky, Ivan. Charles Schepens.

Lancet 2006; 367: 1974.

79   *"Every few weeks"*: Ostrum, Meg. *The Surgeon and the Shepherd: Two Resistance Heroes in Vichy France* (Lincoln, NE; University of Nebraska Press, 2004), 37.

80   *"When I looked inside the patients' eyes"*: Ostrum, *The Surgeon*, 155.

81   *Schepens built this rudimentary prototype*: Albert, Daniel and Diane Edwards, eds. *The History of Ophthalmology* (Cambridge, MA; Blackwell Science 1996), 197.

81   *hit by a V-2 rocket*: William Tasman, M.D. Personal communication, August 8, 2011.

81   *the place to go was America*: Ibid.

81   *Today it is the largest independent eye research institute*: McMeel J, Van de Velde R. In Memoriam Charles L. Schepens M.D. Bull Soc Belge Ophth 2006; 302: 7-8.

81   *success rate of reattachment*: Oransky 1974.

82   *"I did not want to be considered"*: Ostrum, *The Surgeon*, 170.

83   *Primitive early treatments*: Albert, *The History*, 199.

83   *53% success rate*: Ibid., 200.

84   *The vitrector instrument*: Ibid., 201.

Chapter Five | *"…eighteen out of twenty-one…"*
Arnall Patz, Retinopathy of Prematurity, and a Looming Crisis

93   *Arnall Patz, as his friends*: The author thanks Mrs. Ellen Patz, Dr. Patz's widow, for reviewing this chapter and for providing helpful insight into Dr. Patz's personal history and motivation throughout his career.

94   *And it was Brown's father*: Mrs. Ellen Patz. Personal communication, August 18, 2011.

94   *It has been said*: Silverstein A. On presentation of the Friedenwald Memorial Award in Ophthalmology to Arnall Patz. Invest Ophthalmol Vis Sci 1980 Oct; 19(10): 1128.

95   *This disease was the leading*: Patz A. Retrolental Fibroplasia (Retinopathy of Prematurity). Am J Ophthalmol 1982 Oct; 94(4): 552-554.

95   *In those days*: Tasman W, Patz A, McNamara JA, et al. Retinopathy of Prematurity: The Life of a Lifetime Disease. Am J Ophthalmol 2006;

141: 167-174.

95   *Except that Patz realized:* Patz A, Hoeck L, De La Cruz E. Studies of
      the effect of high oxygen administration in retrolental fibroplasia. Am
      J Ophthalmol 1952 Sep; 35(9): 1248-1253. Also, Mrs. Ellen Patz.
      Personal communication, August 18, 2011.

96   *The NIH said:* Goldberg M, McDonnell P. Arnall Patz, MD: Physician,
      Scientist, and Humanitarian. Arch Ophthalmol 2005; 123: 1600-
      1602.

97   *Some of them could not:* Ibid., 1600.

97   *Patz studied the babies:* Patz 1952: 1248-1253.

97   *He also demonstrated:* Patz A. Oxygen Studies in Retrolental Fibroplasia.
      Am J Ophthalmol 1954 Sep; 38(3): 291-308.

98   *He first tried using the opossum:* Mrs. Ellen Patz. Personal communication,
      August 18, 2011.

98   *"On one occasion while":* Tasman 169.

98   *he saw that high oxygen exposure:* Patz 1954: 291-308.

98   *Patz also realized that:* Mrs. Ellen Patz. Personal communication,
      August 18, 2011.

99   *Patz had the satisfaction:* Goldberg 1600-1602.

100   *he downplayed his own contributions:* Tasman 167-174.

101   *In 2004, Patz received:* Ferris F. Arnall Patz, MD. The Spirit of
      Collaboration. Arch Ophthalmol 2010; 128(12): 1602-1603.

102   *there has been a growing crisis:* Wagner R. A Potential Retinopathy of
      Prematurity Crisis. J Pediatr Ophthalmol Strabismus 2002 Nov-Dec;
      39(6): 325. Also, Kemper AR, Freedman SF, Wallace DK. Retinopathy
      of prematurity care: Patterns of care and workforce analysis. J AAPOS
      2008; 12(4): 344-348.

102   *From 1981 to 2008, the rate of premature births:* Jackson K, Scott
      K, Graff Zivin J, et al. Cost-utility analysis of tele-medicine and
      ophthalmoscopy for retinopathy of prematurity management. Arch
      Ophthalmol 2008; 126(4): 493-499.

102   *A 2006 survey:* American Academy of Ophthalmology. Ophthalmol-
      ogists warn of shortage of specialists who treat premature babies with
      blinding eye condition. Eyenet 2006; 10(7): 17-19.

103 *premature babies have a higher incidence of:* Tasman 172.

105 *Similar changes have happened:* Banta JV. Medical liability crisis: an international problem. Developmental Medicine and Child Neurology 2003; 45: 363.

106 *Incidentally, there are approximately:* Berrington de Gonzalez A, Mahesh M, Kim K, et al. Projected cancer risks from computed tomographic scans performed in the United States in 2007. Arch Intern Med 2009; 169(22): 2071-2077.

Chapter Six | *"Whaddya mean it's a shot? In my eye?"*
**Judah Folkman, Angiogenesis, and the Treatment of
Wet Macular Degeneration**

115 *On February 24, 1933:* The author thanks Mrs. Paula Folkman, Dr. Folkman's widow, for reviewing and providing comments on this chapter. The author also acknowledges Robert Cooke's comprehensive biography of Dr. Folkman (Cooke, Robert. *Dr. Folkman's War.* New York; Random House, 2001.) as a valuable resource that provided insight into Dr. Folkman's outlook and motivation through the course of his long career.

115 *Above all, Rabbi Folkman exhorted:* Cooke, Robert. *Dr. Folkman's War* (New York; Random House, 2001), 6.

116 *"In that case":* Ibid., 12.

117 *As a medical student, he developed:* Folkman MJ, Watkins E. An artificial conduction system for the management of experimental complete heart block. Surg Forum 1957; 8: 331-334.

117 *The Navy sent Folkman:* Cooke, *Dr. Folkman's,* 45-49.

118 *They were able to keep thyroid glands healthy:* Folkman MJ, Long DM, Becker FF. Growth and metastasis of tumor in organ culture. Cancer 1963; 16: 453-467.

118 *Folkman and Becker decided to inject:* Cooke, *Dr. Folkman's,* 52-57.

123 *He confirmed what he'd seen before:* Folkman J, Cole P, Zimmerman S. Tumor behavior in isolated perfused organs: in vitro growth and metastases of biopsy material in rabbit thyroid and canine intestinal segment. Ann Surg 1966; 164: 491-502.

124 *Folkman was criticized:* Cooke, *Dr. Folkman's,* 86.

124 *there was a logical counterargument:* Nathan DG, Gimbrone MA. Judah Folkman, M.D. 1933-2008. The Pharos 2009; winter: 7.

125 *First he implanted:* Gimbrone MA, Leapman SB, Cotran RS, Folkman J. Tumor dormancy in vivo by prevention of neovascularization. J Exp Med 1972; 136: 261-276.

125 *He gave the theoretical signal a name:* Folkman J, Merler E, Abernathy C, Williams G. Isolation of a tumor fraction responsible for angiogenesis. J Exp Med 1971; 133: 275-288.

125 *"It has not been appreciated":* Folkman J. Tumor angiogenesis. Therapeutic implications. N Engl J Med 1971; 285: 1182-1186.

126 *"It's theftproof":* Cooke, *Dr. Folkman's,* 105.

126 *"A Harvard surgeon":* Brody, Jane. "Tests Hint Protein is Vital to Cancers." *New York Times,* March 28, 1972: 1.

128 *Some accused Harvard:* Cooke, *Dr. Folkman's,* 146.

128 *"purifying dirt", "You're making a mockery", "Haven't we supported":* Ibid., 117, 183, 182.

128 *Folkman and his associates were able to show:* Folkman J, Haudenschild CC, Zetter BR. Long-term culture of capillary endothelial cells. Proc Natl Acad Sci USA 1979; 76(10): 5217-5221.

128 *Folkman and two associates:* Shing Y, Folkman J, Sullivan R, et al. Heparin affinity: purification of a tumor-derived capillary endothelial cell growth factor. Science 1984; 223: 1296-1298.

129 *a scientist named Napoleone Ferrara:* Cooke, *Dr. Folkman's,* 209-210.

129 *Harold Dvorak, a doctor:* Ibid., 210-211.

129 *One of the first anti-angiogenic agents:* Brouty-Boye D, Zetter BR. Inhibition of cell motility by interferon. Science 1980; 208: 516-518.

129 *In 1994, Folkman's lab isolated:* O'Reilly MS, Holmgren L, Chen C, et al. Angiostatin induces and sustains dormancy of human primary tumors in mice. Nat Med 1996; 2: 689-692.

129 *When they treated with another factor:* O'Reilly MS, Boehm T, Shing Y, et al. Endostatin: an endogenous inhibitor of angiogenesis and tumor growth. Cell 1997; 88: 277-285.

130 *In 2004, bevacizumab:* Hurwitz H, Fehrenbacker L, Novotny W, et al. Bevacizumab plus irinotecan, fluorouracil, and leucovorin for

metastatic colorectal cancer. N Engl J Med 2004; 350: 2335-2342.

130 *In the 1990s, Folkman had inspired a group of ophthalmologists:* Adamis AP, Miller JW, Bernal MT, et al. Increased vascular endothelial growth factor levels in the vitreous of eyes with proliferative diabetic retinopathy. Am J Ophthalmol 1994; 118: 445-450. Also, Adamis AP, Shima DR, Tolentino MJ, et al. Inhibition of vascular endothelial growth factor prevents retinal ischemia-associated iris neovascularization in a nonhuman primate. Arch Ophthalmol 1996; 114: 66-71. And, Miller JW. The Harvard Angiogenesis Story: The Paul Henkind Memorial Lecture. Presented at The Macula Society 34th Annual Meeting. Boca Raton, FL. March 11, 2011.

131 *"[He] persisted in the face of":* Brower V. Judah Folkman leaves expanding legacy. JNCI 2008; 100(6): 380-381.

132 *we have Judah Folkman to thank:* Judah Folkman would have been the first to emphasize that the discoveries made in his lab would not have been possible without the collaboration of many other doctors and scientists. Regrettably, for the sake of this straightforward narrative, and with the general reader in mind, I have not listed the names of all those who made important contributions to help elucidate angiogenesis. Many of their names are found as co-authors of the papers cited for this chapter.

133 *macular degeneration is the leading cause:* Eye Diseases Prevalence Research Group. Prevalence of age-related macular degeneration in the United States. Arch Ophthalmol 2004; 122(4): 564-572.

133 *9.1 million Americans:* Rein DB, Wittenborn BS, Zhang X, et al. Forecasting age-related macular degeneration through the year 2050. Arch Ophthalmol 2009; 127(4): 533.

133 *In a 2008 study of Medicare patients:* Brechner RJ, Rosenfeld PJ, Babish D, et al. Pharmacotherapy for neovascular age-related macular degeneration: an analysis of the 100% 2008 Medicare fee-for-service Part B claims file. Am J Ophthalmol 2011; 151: 887.

135 *Rosenfeld published his results:* Rosenfeld PJ, Moshfeghi AA, Puliafito CA. Optical coherence tomography findings after an intravitreal injection of bevacizumab (Avastin) for neovascular age-related macular degeneration. Ophthalmic Surg Lasers Imaging 2005; 36(4): 331-335. Also, Rich RM, Rosenfeld PJ, Puliafito CA, et al. Short-term safety and efficacy of intravitreal bevacizumab (Avastin) for

neovascular age-related macular degeneration. Retina 2006; 26(5): 495-511.

135 *Genentech sent their president:* Genentech tells a riled AAO reception: Avastin will be available. Review of Ophthalmology 2007 Dec; 14(12): 6.

136 *"Genentech refuses to help":* Associated Press. "Genentech refuses to help study cheaper drug." *The Oregonian,* August 27, 2008.

136 *"Genentech offers secret rebates":* Pollack, Andrew. "Genentech offers secret rebates for eye drug." *New York Times,* November 3, 2010.

136 *"Genentech fights the use of":* Mundy, Alicia, and Jennifer Corbett Dooren. "Genentech fights the use of its own cheaper drug." *Wall Street Journal,* April 28, 2011.

136 *The first-year results:* The CATT Research Group. Ranibizumab and Bevacizumab for neovascular age-related macular degeneration. N Engl J Med 2011; 364(20): 1897-1908.

137 *In 2012, the two-year results:* The CATT Research Group. Ranibizumab and Bevacizumab for neovascular age-related macular degeneration: Two-Year Results. Ophthalmology 2012; 119(7): 1388-1398.

137 *"Health care providers and payers":* Rosenfeld PJ. Bevacizumab versus Ranibizumab for AMD. N Engl J Med 2011; 364(20): 1967.

137 *Rosenfeld also testified:* Philip Rosenfeld testimony at Senate Hearing of the Special Committee on Aging. "A Prescription for Savings: Reducing Drug Costs to Medicare," July 21, 2011. Full text accessed at http://www.fdsys.gov on February 26, 2012.

Chapter Seven | *"I really do want to see the alarm clock in the morning."*
The Evolution of Refractive Surgery

145 *In centuries past:* Bores, Leo. *Refractive Eye Surgery, 2nd ed.* (Malden, MA; Blackwell Science, Inc., 2001), 6.

145 *Dr. J. Ball:* Ibid., 6.

145 *In 1894, Dr. William Bates:* Bates W. A suggestion of an operation to correct astigmatism. Arch Ophthalmol 1894; 23: 9-13.

146 *A Dutch physician:* Lans W. Experimentelle Untersuchungen uber Entstehung von Astigmatismus durch nicht-perforirende cornea-wunden. Graefes Arch Klin Exp Ophthalmol 1898; 45: 117-152.

147 *In 1936, a Japanese ophthalmologist:* Bores, *Refractive Eye,* 191.

147 *In 1939, Sato published:* Sato T. Treatment of conical cornea (incision of Descemet's membrane). Acta Soc Ophthalmol Jpn 1939; 43: 544-555.

147 *His successful results:* Sato T. Crosswise incisions of Descemet's membrane for the treatment of advanced keratoconus. Acta Soc Ophthalmol Jpn 1942; 46: 469-470.

147 *but over time, usually about twenty years after surgery:* Akiyama K, Tanaka M, Kanai A, et al. Problems arising from Sato's radial keratotomy procedure from Japan. CLAO J 1984; 10: 179-184. Also, Beatty RD, Smith RE. Thirty year follow-up of posterior radial keratotomy. Am J Ophthalmol 1987; 103: 330-331. And, Yamaguchi T, Kanai A, Tanaka M, et al. Bullous keratopathy after anterior-posterior radial keratotomy for myopia and myopic astigmatism. Am J Ophthalmol 1982; 93: 600-606.

148 *First published in 1949:* Barraquer JI. Oueratoplasia refractive. Estudios Inform 1949; 2: 10-21.

148 *Leaving the patient on the table:* Reinstein DZ, Archer TJ, Gobbe M. The History of LASIK. J Refract Surg 2012; 28(4): 291-293.

148 *He called his technique:* Barraquer JI. Keratomileusis for the correction of myopia. Arch Soc Am Oftal Optom 1964; 5: 27-48.

148 *a Russian ophthalmologist named:* Tannebaum S. Svyatoslav Fyodorov, M.D. Innovative eye surgeon. J Amer Optom Asso 1995; 66(10): 652-654.

149 *"If a fist can do this":* Bores, *Refractive Eye,* 198.

149 *Fyodorov's incisions weakened:* Fyodorov SN, Durnev W. Operation of dosaged dissection of corneal circular ligament in cases of myopia of mild degree. Ann Ophthalmol 1979; 11: 1885-1890.

150 *This repetitive method was considered very successful:* Durnev W. Characteristics of surgical correction of myopia after 16 and 32 peripheral anterior radial non-perforating incisions. In: Fyodorov SN, ed. *Surgery of anomalies in ocular refraction* (Moscow; The Moscow Research Institute of Ocular Microsurgery, 1981), 33-35.

151 *a doctor named Leo Bores:* Bores LD. Radial keratotomy. A safe, effective way to correct a handicap. Surv Ophthalmol 1983; 28: 101-105.

151 *others called him a "buccaneer":* Bores, *Refractive Eye,* xv.

151   *The National Eye Institute initiated:* Waring G, Lynn M, Gelender H, et al. Results of prospective evaluation of radial keratotomy (PERK) study one year after surgery. Ophthalmology 1985; 92: 177-196.

152   *Even at the height of its popularity:* Deitz M, Sanders D, Marks R. Radial keratotomy – an overview of the Kansas city study. Ophthalmology 1984; 91: 467-477.

152   *not as stable as previously thought:* Waring G, Lynn M, McDonnell R. Results of the Prospective Evaluation of Radial Keratotomy (PERK) Study 10 years after surgery. Arch Ophthalmol 1994; 112: 1298-1308.

152   *A Russian physicist named:* Reinstein 294.

153   *In 1981, an engineer named:* Ibid., 294.

153   *In 1983, Trokel and Srinivasan:* Trokel SL, Srinivasan R, Schubert HD. Excimer laser surgery of the cornea. Am J Ophthalmol 1983; 96: 710-715. Also, Krueger RR, Trokel SL, Schubert HD. Interaction of ultraviolet laser light with the cornea. Invest Ophthalmol Vis Sci 1985; 26(11): 1455-1464.

153   *In 1985, a German ophthalmologist named:* Seiler T, Wollensak J. In vivo experiments with the excimer laser: technical parameters and healing processes. Ophthalmologica 1986; 192: 65-70. Also, Krueger RR, Rabinowitz YS, Binder PS. The 25th Anniversary of Excimer Lasers in Refractive Surgery: Historical Review. J Refract Surg 2010; 26 (10): 753. And, Reinstein 296.

153   *In 1988, Dr. Marguerite McDonald:* Kreuger 2010: 754. Also, McDonald MB, Kaufman HE, Frantz JM, et al. Excimer laser ablation in a human eye. Arch Ophthalmol 1989; 107: 641-642.

153   *The method was patented:* Peyman G. History of LASIK. Ophthalmol 2007; 114(7): 1414.

153   *Greek surgeon Ioannis Pallikaris:* Pallikaris IG, Papatzanaki ME, Stathi EZ, et al. Laser in situ keratomileusis. Lasers Surg Med 1990; 10: 463-468.

154   *In 2010, it was estimated that:* Reinstein 291.

154   *The collective dreams:* Many additional scientists and physicians contributed to the evolution of refractive surgery. Unfortunately, it is not possible to include all of them in this narrative. Some of their names can be found in the citations listed for this chapter.

156 *By 2008, this had been reduced to:* American Academy of Ophthalmology: Historical Payments for Cataract CPT Codes, prepared for June 2011.

158 *"Just feed the patient's refraction into the computer":* Bores, *Refractive Eye,* 385.

158 *Such self-promotion:* Frayer, William C. *An Ophthalmic Journey: Fifty Years at the University of Pennsylvania* (Philadelphia, PA; Scheie Eye Institute, 2002), 75.

Chapter Eight | *"If I cannot discover a way to read and write… I shall kill myself."*

Louis Braille and Nightwriting

163 *"As [Jesus] went along":* The Holy Bible, John 9: 1-3. New International version.

164 *Paris 1821:* This dramatized account of Braille's life at the Institute for Blind Youth is drawn from the biographical texts and articles cited below. Though these events could have occurred in the manner described, they are fictional.

168 *Only three!:* Neimark, Anne E. *Touch of Light: The Story of Louis Braille* (New York; Harcourt, Brace & World, Inc., 1970), 78.

169 *the blind boys couldn't see each other cry:* Ibid., 79.

170 *"I called it nightwriting":* Sakula A. That the blind may read: the legacy of Valentin Haüy, Charles Barbier, Louis Braille, and William Moon. J Med Biography 1998; 6: 23.

172 *As a toddler:* How Louis Braille Lost His Sight. Sightsaving Review: official publication of the National Society for the Prevention of Blindness 1952; 22(4): 219.

172 *his father walked outside:* Bryant Jennifer F. *Louis Braille: Teacher of the Blind* (New York; Chelsea House Publishers, 1994), 29.

172 *Many authors have considered:* Freedman, Russell. *Out of Darkness: The Story of Louis Braille* (New York; Clarion Books, 1997), 5-8. Also, Neimark, *Touch of Light,* 11-17.

172 *probably an awl:* Braille Centenary. Lancet 1952; 1(6721): 1248. Also, Bryant, *Louis Braille,* 29.

172 *What is certain:* Coltat, Hippolyte. Inauguration du buste de Louis Braille, 1853, 14. Author's note: this is one of the earliest accounts of

the event that blinded Louis Braille, written by his friend and classmate Hippolyte Coltat in 1853. Coltat wrote that Braille's accident was self-inflicted and occurred in his father's workshop with a sharp tool. However, unlike some common versions of the story, Coltat believed that Louis' father was beside him when the injury occurred, and that the offending instrument was a serpette (a knife with a curved blade). Because there are no eyewitness accounts, nor written accounts from the time Braille lived, we cannot be certain of the true details of his injury.

173 *Today, we believe that most likely:* Jimenez K, Olea J, Torres J. Biography of Louis Braille and Invention of the Braille Alphabet. Surv Ophthalmol 2009; 54: 142-149.

173 *His father built him a cane:* Bryant, *Louis Braille,* 35.

173 *One man took a special interest:* Mellor, Michael. *Louis Braille: A touch of genius* (Boston; National Braille Press, 2006), 24. Also, Bryant, *Louis Braille,* 40-41.

174 *The schoolmaster said yes:* Mellor, *Louis Braille,* 25.

174 *The priest had heard of a special school:* Bryant, *Louis Braille,* 44-45.

175 *The captain's dot method had several drawbacks:* Ibid., 69.

176 *Braille divided the alphabet systematically:* Ibid., 72-73. Also, Mellor, *Louis Braille,* 62-64.

176 *"Time has lost her wintry gear":* Neimark, *Touch of Light,* 138.

177 *Braille's first setback:* Bryant, *Louis Braille,* 70-71.

178 *"If my eyes will not tell me":* Ibid., 71.

178 *decided to petition France's Interior Minister:* Ibid., 76-77.

179 *many of them opposed:* Bullock JD, Galst JM. The Story of Louis Braille. Arch Ophthalmol 2009; 127(11): 1532-1533.

179 *He developed amazing reading speed:* Bryant, *Louis Braille,* 84.

179 *"his method gave us the first idea":* Freedman, *Out of Darkness,* 55.

179 *the old director was ousted:* Mellor, *Louis Braille,* 97-98.

180 *Dufau himself had invented:* Ibid., 99.

180 *Dufau banned the dot system:* Ibid., 99.

181 *he had ordered all the books:* Bryant, *Louis Braille,* 95.

181 *He became the first sighted person:* Bickel, Lennard. *Triumph Over Darkness: The Life of Louis Braille* (Anstey, Leicestershire; F.A. Thorpe Publishing, 1988), 269.

182 *Dufau came around to Guadet's reasoning.* Bryant, *Louis Braille*, 99-100.

182 *on February 22, 1844:* Ibid., 102-104. Also, Freedman, *Out of Darkness,* 71-72.

184 *"...we, the blind, are":* "Helen Keller Pays Tribute to Braille." *New York Times,* June 22, 1952: 20.

184 *His hands, however:* Sakula 24.

Chapter Nine
Visionaries

199 *patients have been able to distinguish:* Ahuja AK, Dorn JD, Caspi A, et al. Blind subjects implanted with the Argus II retinal prosthesis are able to improve performance in a spatial-motor task. Br J Ophthalmol 2011; 95(4): 539-543. Also, Dorn JD, Ahuja AK, Caspi A, et al. The detection of motion by blind subjects with the epiretinal 60-electrode (Argus II) retinal prosthesis. Arch Ophthalmol 2013; 131(2): 183-189.

199 *restored some sight to blind dogs:* Acland GM, Aguirre GD, Ray J, et al. Gene therapy restores vision in a canine model of childhood blindness. Nat Genet 2001; 28(1): 92-95. Also, Maguire AM, Simonelli F, Pierce EA, et al. Safety and efficacy of gene transfer for Leber's congenital amaurosis. N Engl J Med 2008; 358(21): 2240-2248.

200 *researchers have demonstrated success:* Kokkinaki M, Sahibxada N, Golestaneh N. Human induced pluripotent stem-derived retinal pigment epithelium (RPE) cells exhibit ion transport, membrane potential, polarized vascular endothelial growth factor secretion, and gene expression pattern similar to native RPE. Stem Cells 2011; 29: 825-835.

SELECTED BIBLIOGRAPHY

Albert, Daniel and Diane Edwards, eds. *The History of Ophthalmology.* Cambridge, MA; Blackwell Science, 1996.

Apple, David J. *Sir Harold Ridley and His Fight for Sight.* Thorofare, NJ; Slack, 2006.

Bickel, Lennard. *Triumph Over Darkness: The Life of Louis Braille.* Anstey, Leicestershire; F.A. Thorpe Publishing, 1988.

Bryant Jennifer F. *Louis Braille: Teacher of the Blind.* New York; Chelsea House Publishers, 1994.

Bores, Leo. *Refractive Eye Surgery, 2nd ed.* Malden, MA; Blackwell Science, Inc., 2001.

Cooke, Robert. *Dr. Folkman's War.* New York; Random House, 2001.

Frayer, William C. *An Ophthalmic Journey: Fifty Years at the University of Pennsylvania.* Philadelphia, PA; Scheie Eye Institute, 2002.

Freedman, Russell. *Out of Darkness: The Story of Louis Braille.* New York; Clarion Books, 1997.

Kelman, Charles D. *Through My Eyes: The story of a surgeon who dared to take on the medical world*. New York; Crown, 1985.

Korda, Michael. *With Wings Like Eagles: The Untold Story of the Battle of Britain*. New York, NY; Harper Perennial, 2009.

Mellor, Michael. *Louis Braille: A touch of genius*. Boston; National Braille Press, 2006.

Neimark, Anne E. *Touch of Light: The Story of Louis Braille*. New York; Harcourt, Brace & World, Inc., 1970.

Ostrum, Meg. *The Surgeon and the Shepherd: Two Resistance Heroes in Vichy France*. Lincoln, NE; University of Nebraska Press, 2004.

ABOUT THE AUTHOR

Andrew Lam, M.D., was born in Philadelphia and raised in central Illinois. He graduated *summa cum laude* in history from Yale University, then attended medical school at the University of Pennsylvania. He subsequently completed his specialty training in ophthalmology and retina surgery at the Wills Eye Hospital in Philadelphia, where he served as a chief resident. Dr. Lam has authored numerous scientific articles and is currently an Assistant Professor of Ophthalmology at Tufts University School of Medicine. He resides in western Massachusetts with his wife and four children.

CPSIA information can be obtained
at www.ICGtesting.com
Printed in the USA
BVHW031410220323
660920BV00004B/436

9 781617 203794